You *Can* Prevent Cancer

Dr. Michael Colgan
with Lesley Colgan, MS

Apple Publishing
Vancouver, BC
2007

*This book is not intended for the treatment of disease, nor as a substitute for medical
treatment, nor as an alternative to medical advice. It is a review of scientific evidence
presented for information purposes, to increase public knowledge of developments in
the field of cancer prevention. Although the information contained in this book was
prepared from sources that are believed to be accurate and reliable, the publisher
strongly advises readers to seek the advice of their personal health care professional(s)
before proceeding with any changes in _any_ health care program.*

Includes bibliographical references and index.
ISBN 978-1-896817-07-1

**1. Cancer--Prevention--Popular works. 2. Cancer--Nutritional
Aspect--Popular works. 3. Cancer--Exercise-therap--Popular works. 1. Title.**

RC268.45.C64 2007   616.99'4052   C2006-906779-1

Printed in Hong Kong

Apple Tree Publishing Ltd
Vancouver, Canada

To My Girls,
Megan and Tammy

Acknowledgements

The work of many fine researchers elevates this book. Many have personally encouraged me to make a new public accounting of the battle against cancer. I hope I have done you all justice.

Help I had aplenty. With her constant support and enthusiasm, unfailing humor, incisive analysis, and meticulous editing, my executive, Brenda Kennedy, has kept me from losing my head throughout the frantic time of writing. Warm thanks go also to my assistant, Eva Boucek, for her calm and resourceful help in preparation of the manuscript, cover design, and other tasks too numerous to mention. Thanks also to Nolan Machan of Apple Publishing for his boundless enthusiasm and prompt responses to everything I asked.

With her wonderful zest for life, my dear, incomparable partner Lesley did much of the research for this book and again took on most of my job, in addition to her own, in order to give me the freedom to write. This book has been bubbling in my brain for the last three years. She has given it the chance to pour out.

Despite all of this help, or perhaps because of it, the conclusions herein remain on my head alone.

Introduction

Through papers, correspondence, personal meetings, and lectures that were highlights of my early career, I had the good fortune to learn from Roger Williams, Linus Pauling, Hans Selye, Richard Feynman, and Jonas Salk to become a relentless seeker after truth. Other great scientists, too many to name, also assisted me and continue to assist me in this quest which is now in its 33rd year.

I am a scientist, not a physician. My expertise is in research, analyzing the results of research, and figuring out the implications of these results for human health. My first book on cancer in 1989 led tens of thousands of people to my door, seeking counsel. Back then it was not a happy cavalcade. Sometimes I was able to give them and their physicians new information that influenced the course of their disease, and often people adopted sensible prevention strategies which reduced their risk of some cancers and eliminated their risk of others. But in the '80s and early '90s, scientific knowledge of cancer was somewhat basic compared with the science of today.

In the first decade of this century we have learned more about cancer than in all previous history. Using current research, it is now possible to construct extremely effective strategies for cancer prevention. It is not a matter of public health policy which always seems to lag a decade behind the research. It is a matter of personal knowledge and the personal decision to protect yourself. Many thousands of individuals have taken this decision, with the result that cancer death rates are now falling for the first time since I was born, and that is beginning to be a very long time ago.

Join me in the quest to defeat the cancer enemy, an enemy that causes far more unnecessary deaths every year than all the terrorists, wars, tsunamis, hurricanes, floods, and earthquakes put together. Unlike the treachery of warmongers and the unpredictability of natural disasters, the parameters of most cancers are now known, allowing us to construct virtually impenetrable armor against them.

Michael Colgan
Colgan Institute
Saltspring Island
British Columbia
1 July 2006

Table of CONTENTS

1

The War On Cancer

Good news. When I wrote my first book on cancer prevention in 1989, it was the grimmest complex of diseases.[1] Chances of a cure were less than 50%. Cancer rates were rising rapidly, with little understanding of why and no relief in sight. Now in 2006, the picture is getting a lot brighter. Here's how it happened.

With the National Cancer Act of 1971, President Richard Nixon declared a knock-down, drag-out *"War On Cancer."* Billions of tax dollars were allocated, and the people believed cancer would be beaten – *fast*. Every year afterwards, the US National Cancer Institute claimed great progress. Almost daily, media reports cited shrinking tumors, better drugs, targeted radiation, and a host of other triumphs of advanced medicine. By the mid-1980s, after 15 years of the *"War,"* it became obvious that most of these claims concerned winning small skirmishes, while utterly losing the battle.

The True Face of Cancer: 1970 -1995

In May 1986, cancer specialists John Bailar, then of the Harvard School of Public Health, and Eileen Smith of the University of Iowa published meticulous research in the *New England Journal of Medicine* showing that cancer survival had not improved at all.[2] As shown in Figure 1.1, they found that cancer death rates **steadily increased** from 1960 into the 1980s.

Apologists for big-business cancer medicine rushed to claim that cancer only seemed to be an increasing problem because the American population was growing older. Older people are more subject to cancer than young people. The higher numbers of elderly patients therefore inflated the cancer figures. Codswallop!

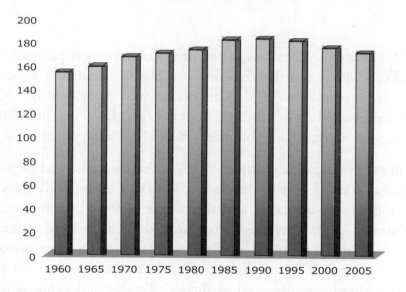

Figure 1.1. US cancer death rates per 100,000 population from all cancers combined, 1960-2005. Adapted by the Colgan Institute from Bailar 1986[2] and US National Cancer Institute figures to June 2006.[3]

In February 1994, a government research team led by Devra Davis of the US Department of Health and Human Services published their analysis of the latest cancer figures in the *Journal of the American Medical Association*. Men of the baby-boomer generation, then only in their 40s and 50s, suffered nearly *three times* the cancer rate their grandfathers did at the same ages. Women baby-boomers had 30% more cancers overall than their grandmothers, and more than *twice* the rate of breast cancer.[4]

Cancer Treatment Failure

What about the wonders of modern chemotherapy still being touted almost daily in the media? Eminent medical biostatistician Ulrich Abel spent a year analyzing the efficacy of all forms of chemotherapy against all types of epithelial cancers. Epithelial cancers encompass all common cancers and account for 80% of our cancer deaths.

Abel did not find many cures. Instead he found that most clinical trials claim success when the therapy causes tumors to shrink. In many forms of cancer, however, tumors are merely one of the symptoms of an underlying systemic disease. Shrinkage or even disappearance of tumors still leaves the disease intact. That's why so many cancers recur. A tumor is much like Osama bin Laden, the obvious sign of a network of evil which cannot be destroyed simply by cutting him out.

Most important, after meticulously reviewing thousands of studies, Abel concluded in 1990 that,

> *There is no evidence for the majority of cancers, that treatment with these drugs exerts any positive influence on survival or*

quality of life in patients with advanced disease.[5]

Another nail in the coffin comes from oncologists who treat patients with chemotherapy. Abel cites poll after poll of cancer physicians, showing that many would refuse chemotherapy if they developed cancer themselves.[5]

For most cancers, chemotherapy has hardly improved at all. By 1996, the prestigious British medical journal *Lancet* had published a review, representative of cancer specialists worldwide, by molecular biologist and chemotherapy specialist Michael Sporn of Dartmouth University, New Hampshire. Professor Sporn concluded that the followers of the National Cancer Institute had an obsession with trying to cure advanced cancer that simply had not worked.[6]

It still doesn't work. Leading cancer specialist Guy Faquet of the Medical College of Georgia has published over 100 studies on cancer, largely funded by the US National Cancer Institute. In an impeccably documented new book in late 2005, Professor Faquet blasted chemotherapy. His conclusion:

While most patients achieve some degree of tumor response, few survive longer as a result.[7]

Appalled by the real picture of cancer in the early 1990s, many researchers refocused their attention. They turned away from chemotherapy and radiation treatments that were doing little for well-established cancers, and toward early diagnosis and cure of pre-cancerous conditions, and especially ***prevention of cancer***. It has made all the difference.

The Good News

As a 21-year survivor of cancer myself, I am so pleased to report the latest cancer figures for the US, released on the 19th of February, 2006. They show that total deaths by cancer in 2003 were 369 fewer than in 2002, even with the 3 million increase in the US population.[8, 9] Not a great number, but the first time it has happened in my lifetime.

It's important because death is the only sure measure. I believe firmly that I survived cancer because of my nutrition program, but as a scientist, I can't be sure. We can argue endlessly about survivorship, tumor disappearance, better quality of life, but after a couple of days, you have to admit to a corpse that the treatment just isn't working. When deaths decline, we *know* we are getting somewhere.

There's even better news. On the 5th of October, 2005, the Director of the National Cancer Institute, Andrew von Eschenhbach, announced the latest analysis, showing that overall annual death rates from cancer in America have been falling by about 1% per year since 1995.[8, 9] One percent doesn't seem a lot, but it represents tens of thousands of people saved from cancer.

More than half of all cancer deaths are caused by just four types of cancer: prostate, colorectal, lung, and breast cancer. Collectively, the Big Four are expected to kill about 290,000 Americans in 2006. Overall, cancer deaths are expected to hit 565,000.[10] Just a 1% win in the cancer war saves about 5,650 Americans from death every year, more than all the efforts for all the years against terrorists.

We are starting to win big battles. Prostate cancer death rates have fallen 4% per year since 1994. Colorectal cancer death rates have fallen 2% per year. Breast cancer death rates have fallen in men, but sadly not in women. I suggest some potent strategies to reduce female breast cancer ahead.

The best news is for lung cancer, the greatest cause by far of cancer death in both men and women. Lung cancer is expected to kill 162,500 Americans in 2006, and to spawn 175,000 new cases.[6] Over the last five years, however, death rates have declined for all the top 10 lung cancers in men, and for 9 of the top 10 lung cancers in women.[8-10]

Little of this decline happened because of better treatments. Almost all of it occurred because of fewer cases. It happened because of cancer prevention – mainly, prevention of smoke.

During the 1990s, the deceit of the tobacco industry was at last successfully condemned in the courts. Legions of smokers were finally convinced that ingesting tobacco smoke is an inevitable, unbeatable cause of lung cancer. Adults, especially those aged 20 – 39, quit smoking in droves, or never started. And many thousands prevented lung cancer by refusing to work or play in the disease-bearing fug of second-hand smoke.

The CEO of the American Cancer Society, John Seffrin, states:

> *Declines in mortality rates from many tobacco-related cancers in men, represent an important, but incomplete, triumph of public health in the 21st century.*[9]

I disagree. As explained in Chapter 3 ahead, it's **not** public health that deserves the accolade. It's all the individuals who made the personal decision to prevent cancer themselves.

When will the scaliwags of American health politics realize that, in a face-to-face battle with cancer, all the high-tech medical weaponry is virtually powerless? Cancer infiltrates by stealth, and usually exposes its head as a tumor only after it owns the body. Then it matters hardly a whit that the head is chopped off. The only way to defeat cancer is to build an impenetrable defence.

I advocated in the 1980s that there was about a 90% chance of preventing cancer if you did everything perfectly.[1] Today the odds have swung further in your favor. You, by your own actions, can create a superb strategy to avoid this terrible complex of diseases, better than any doctor, any hospital, any medical system on Earth.

You can provide your body with a nearly invincible suit of armor against cancer by using recent discoveries in medical science. You don't have to be a rocket scientist to understand them. They are straightforward and convenient for lifetime use by everyone. You can start today to remove almost all the risks of cancer from your life.

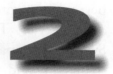

Prevention, Prevention

The answer to all major cancers lies not in surgery, chemotherapy, radiation, or any other kind of medical treatment. These procedures, though useful for treatment once the disease is established, have such a high failure rate that we have to find a better way. New science has now pinpointed the cancer answer. It lies all around you, in your food, your lifestyle, and your environment.

If it seems too good to be true, consider. In July 2000, the prestigious medical journal, the *New England Journal of Medicine*, published a most important research paper. The study was a collaborative effort of many cancer specialists, led by Paul Lichtenstein of the famed Karolinska Institute in Stockholm, Sweden. Many scientists, including me, had been waiting for it for decades. There were smaller studies, but this was the big one.

After careful planning for years, this research on twins aimed to answer, once and for all, the vital ***nature versus nurture*** question: how much of cancer is caused by genetic factors, which are largely beyond our control, and how much is caused by environment and lifestyle? The researchers followed 44,788 pairs of twins in Sweden, Denmark, and Finland to assess the relative contribution of heredity and environment for eleven different kinds of cancer.

In ***all*** cases, heredity turned out to be the minor cause. There was a heredity component for the Big Four – lung, prostate, breast, and colorectal cancers – with prostate cancer leading at 42% genetically influenced. Lung, breast, and colorectal cancers all have about a 33% genetic influence, but uterine and cervical cancers practically none at all. Results of the twin study are shown in Figure 2.1.

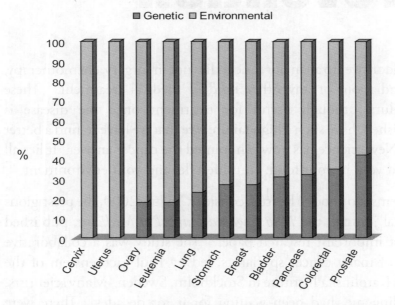

Figure 2.1. Percentage risk of cancer that is genetic and hard to deal with, versus risk that is environmental and can be eliminated. Adapted by the Colgan Institute from Lichtenstein 2001.[1]

The researchers concluded,

> *This finding indicates that the environment has the principal role in causing cancer.*[1]

Following this study and other new research, in September 2001 the Karolinska Institute published a consensus by leading cancer specialists worldwide, stating that most cancers are caused by environmental and lifestyle factors within our power to modify.[2] Most cancers, therefore, are preventable.

In the United States, Robert Hoover of the US National Cancer Institute also weighed in:

> *From this work has come the widely accepted estimate that 80-90% of human cancer is due to environmental factors.*[3]

European cancer specialists quickly agreed and published confirming data. The *European Journal of Cancer* compared the large reductions in cancer deaths resulting from cancer prevention programs that target environmental causes, with reductions in deaths resulting from advances in cancer treatment. Prevention won hands down!

Simple prevention strategies reduced cancer deaths by 13%, while all the touted breakthroughs in treatment, early diagnosis, screening, etc., reduced deaths by only 6%. The researchers predicted that effective application of prevention could reduce the cancer death rate by a whopping 29% by 2020, whereas advances in treatment would achieve only 4%.[2] Prevention is the way to go!

Yet even with this certain knowledge today, only 1% of cancer dollars are spent on prevention. Virtually all the billions taken from your taxes for cancer are spent on treatments and administration, much of it ineffective, all of it wildly expensive. Think hard about protecting yourself from cancer before putting your hand in your pocket to support this cancer industry.

Medical science is not focused on prevention of cancer because it is almost impossible to get research grants for it. Unlike a tumor to cut out, you can't see prevention. It earns no fat fees, sells no drugs, confers no status, hones no surgical skills, plumps no resumes, buys no publicity, provides no immediate gratification at all. No researcher or agency can convincingly claim the credit for prevention. Few, therefore, are motivated to try.

Prevention happens slowly, by education, by the dissemination of information that each of us can use for ourselves. Prevention happens when you realize that no physician, hospital, or government agency can protect you against cancer. You have to learn to protect yourself.

Remember, nobody dies of old age. You die of disease of one kind or another, usually of multiple kinds. Nobody becomes a feeble, medically-dependent geriatric because of the passage of time. They become that way because of degenerative processes that have been growing silently in their bodies for many years, as bodily defenses become less and less able to fight the traumas of lifestyle and environment. Cancer is predominantly a lifetime degenerative process. Most cancers grow undetected for decades, before being discovered. Cancer does not grow at all in healthy bodies.

Before you can develop cancer, your body has to lose or damage many of its defense mechanisms. In the healthy person, leading a healthy lifestyle, these mechanisms destroy cancer cells every day without any difficulty at all. Esteemed British scientist and physician Sir Peter Medewar was fond of saying in lectures that the average person gets cancer a million times in life. The healthy body destroys every one of these budding cancers long before they become established.

Today in 2006, cancer is still the second biggest cause of death and infirmity in Western Society. Yet the risk factors for 95% of all cancers are known. Since publication of my first cancer prevention book in 1990,[4] science has learned many novel strategies to counter almost all of them. If you seize this new knowledge presented herein and use it well, you will eliminate the risk of almost all cancers. I hope the evidence presented convinces you to do it.

First, Eliminate the Big Risks

So many things are shown to cause cancer today, from the chlorine in tap water to pesticides on our fruit and vegetables, that many people just give up trying to fight it. It's hard to know what constitutes a real risk and what is just hearsay or media hype. Focused on circulation profits and audience share rather than human health, the media have us running scared at tiny risks of cancer, such as cell phones or microwave-oven emissions, while often failing to stress the big ones.

To many people, for example, pesticides seem to pose a far greater cancer risk than being overweight. In fact, the reverse is true. Cancer risk from overweight is many times that of all the pesticides in our food put together. So the first step in prevention of this dread disease, is to sort the elephants from the fleas.

Despite decades of obfuscation by the tobacco industry, overwhelming evidence shows that smoking (and second-hand smoke) is the biggest cancer risk. Smoking accounts for about

33% of all US cancers and 90% of all US lung cancers.[5]

The second biggest cancer risk is overweight and inactivity, which accounts for 25% of all cancers.[6] These are two different risks to be sure, but occur together so frequently that it's difficult to put separate numbers on them.

The third biggest cancer risk is poor nutrition, which accounts for 16% of all cancers. For most types of cancer, the quarter of the US population eating the fewest fruits and vegetables has twice the cancer rate as the quarter of the population eating the most fruits and vegetables.[7]

Since the turn of the millenium, science has confirmed that the fourth biggest cancer risk is chronic infections. Hepatitis, for example, readily develops into liver cancer. Papilloma viruses are the predominant cause of cervical cancer. Virtually all cervical cancer biopsies contain a papilloma virus of one kind or another.[7,8] Pretty easy to prevent. I cover these and other infection risks for cancer ahead.

A Risk Index to Live By

The Colgan Institute gets numerous requests from individuals and organizations to apportion the degree of risk for different carcinogens. It is a difficult task. Table 2.1 presents our best estimates to date.

Our risk table is based on figures to May 2006 from the National Cancer Institute, the American Cancer Society, from cancer expert Bruce Ames of the University of California (Berkeley), from British cancer experts Richard Doll and Richard Peto, and many others, plus our 33 years of computer records of the major studies.

Table 2.1. The Relative Risks for Cancer

Avoidable Causes of Cancer	% of US Cancer Deaths
Smoking (includes chewing tobacco & second-hand smoke)	33%
Obesity and inactivity	25%
Nutrient deficits and poor diet	16%
Chronic viruses and other infections	7%
Environmental pollution in foods, air and water	5%
Sunlight	2%
Prescription drugs	2%
Illicit drugs and excess alcohol	1%
Radon gas	1%
Radiation	1%
Unavoidable Causes of Cancer	**% of US Cancer Deaths**
Genetic defects	2%
Unknown causes	5%

© Colgan Institute 2006

The table indicates the order in which we believe you should tackle risks of cancer. It makes it clear that a smoker who worries more about environmental pollution is being idiotic. A mother who stuffs her children with high-fat chips and dips, yet refuses to buy apples because they may contain traces of pesticides, is sadly ignorant. And a person who eats the average American diet, but plasters on the sunscreen to prevent skin cancer, has no idea where the big cancers lie.

Successful prevention of cancer is a numbers game. Played well, it allows you to eliminate 93% of all cancer risks. Even playing the game only moderately by not smoking, not associating with smokers, eating an anti-cancer diet, keeping your body fat at a minimum, avoiding pollution, and using the right nutrient supplements, you can avoid 80% of all cancers.

You don't have to live like a monk. I often bet against the 2% cancer risk from sunlight in order to swim at the beach, and the 1% risk from alcohol in order to enjoy wine with dinner. But I wouldn't bet against the 33% risk from smoking, or the 25% risk from being overweight and sedentary. For successful prevention of cancer, first avoid the elephants.

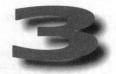

No Smoke
Without Cancer

S moking heads the list as the biggest single risk factor for cancer. Tobacco is the leading avoidable cause of cancer in America, accounting for a whopping one-third of all cancer deaths.[1]

Lung cancer, the most common cancer caused by smoking, is fatal in over 80% of cases.[2] And of the 20% of folk who survive lung cancer, many are non-smokers who have developed the disease from other causes. Lung cancer caused by smoking exhibits a unique, mostly irreversible cell-mutation pattern, not found in lung cancer in non-smokers.[3] Lung cancer from smoking is much more virulent and kills almost all its victims.

Being exposed to second-hand smoke is almost as bad as puffing away yourself. Epidemiological studies show a strong causal association between the risk of lung cancer and exposure to environmental tobacco smoke. Studies of women who are lifelong

non-smokers show that they have a 24% increased risk of lung cancer if their spouse is a smoker. This risk increases with the number of cigarettes smoked and the duration of the marriage.[4]

Other Diseases, Too

You risk a lot more than lung cancer from smoking. Tobacco use is now linked with some 40 diseases.[5] Here we will look at just your risk of various kinds of cancer.

First, smoking increases your risk of squamous cell carcinoma of the head and neck. A recent representative study examined Swedish men aged 40–79. Researchers compared 605 cases and 756 controls in two geographic regions. Those who were tobacco smokers at the time of the study had a greater risk of head and neck cancer. After cessation of smoking, the risk gradually declined, but it took 20 years of non-smoking for the risk to decline to that of the non-smoking population.[6]

Smoking also causes stomach cancer. Another recent study analysed 331 cases and 622 controls over 5 years.[7] The researchers found that smoking doubled the risk for stomach cancer. In those who quit smoking, it took 15 years before their risk dropped to that of non-smokers.

Among women, smoking increases the risk of cervical dysplasia.[8] And if the number of cigarettes exceeds 20 per day, the risk of cervical cancer increases ***five-fold***.[9]

Marijuana, Too

It's not just tobacco smoking that puts you at risk for cancer. Increases in the prevalence of marijuana smoking, especially in young people, have prompted researchers to examine health effects more closely.

One recent study looked at mutations of lymphocytes in marijuana smokers compared with non-smokers. The weed-puffers' immune systems were mutating rapidly.[10] Newborns of marijuana smokers also had significantly higher levels of mutations than newborns of nonsmokers. These cell mutations are pre-cancerous damage to the body that easily develops into cancer.

A further recent study examined both marijuana and cocaine smoking.[11] It found that smokers of any one substance, or of two or more substances (including tobacco), exhibited specific damage in bronchial tissue not found in non-smokers. This damage is a warning sign that often develops into lung cancer.

The Tobacco Industry

Don't believe the insidious hypocrisy of tobacco manufacturers and their henchmen who deny the hundreds of studies like those reviewed above. Well convinced by the evidence, in 1994 the state of Minnesota filed suit against the tobacco industry. Documents released in that trial were the first to reveal that the tobacco industry knew, and internally acknowledged for decades, the disease potential of smoking.[12]

The defendants also knew that nicotine is an addictive drug, and that cigarettes are the ultimate nicotine delivery device. They knew that nicotine addiction can be perpetuated and enhanced through manipulations of cigarette design, and had deliberately carried out those manipulations.[12] Since that trial, multiple states have filed and won lawsuits against the tobacco industry.

What about all those so-called "reduced yield" cigarettes which have lower tar and nicotine (as measured by tobacco company machines)? A review of the research studies done in both America and Britain was published by the American Cancer Society in December 2001. The review concludes,

> *...lung cancer risk continued to increase among older smokers from the 1950s to the 1980s, despite the widespread adoption of lower yield cigarettes.*[13]

'Nuff said!

You Can't Dodge the Bullet

I've heard it a hundred times. "I'm in great shape, Doc. A few ciggies won't hurt." Don't you believe it. Good nutrition, regular exercise and fitness cannot protect you if you continue to smoke.

My saddest example is the late Yul Brynner who always kept his body in superb condition. He ate the best nutrition and exercised vigorously. His one problem was smoking. He smoked all his adult life. He gave it up only when he learned he had developed lung cancer. Too late! Despite the best treatment in the world, he died miserably at the height of his career.

It's never too late to stop smoking if you do so before you get cancer. Just one year after you quit, lung cancer risk is reduced by 50%. In 15 years, it is likely that your lungs will recover completely.

Quitting Smoking

Some researchers put nicotine on the same level as cocaine for its power to addict the human mind. We know that both these drugs stimulate the dopamine system of the **substantia nigra** and the central part of the **hypothalamus** of the brain shown in Figure 3.1. These structures are part of the ancient evolution of the brain that mediates feelings of pleasure and comfort. To a lesser extent, the chemical phenethylamine in chocolate has the same effect.

Tobacco and cocaine are both readily absorbed through the olfactory epithelium of the nose and enter the brain directly when inhaled, which is why cigarettes (and crack pipes) are the most efficient method of delivery. The almost instant buzz of ease from a cigarette as nicotine stimulates the dopamine axis of the brain makes it very difficult to quit smoking.

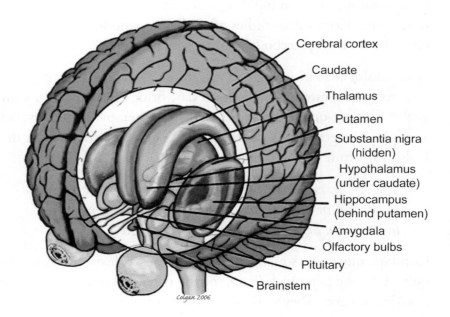

Figure 3.1. Window on the interior of the human brain, showing the position of ancient structures: the substantia nigra and hypothalamus.

Unlike opium and heroin, where quitting triggers very nasty withdrawal syndromes, quitting smoking doesn't make you sick. There is, however, some depression of dopamine function, which can cause depression, fatigue, or anxiety. In some folk, the antidepressant drug **buproprion**, which stimulates the dopamine axis, is an effective crutch for quitting. For most smokers trying to stop, however, buproprion or other antidepressants just don't work.

Some turn to herbs, Oriental medicine, hypnosis, or acupuncture therapies, which offer numerous and varied stop-smoking programs. One currently advertised program "as seen on TV," claims it is "designed to work in seven days." If you believe that, I have some lovely swamp...I mean building lots... in Florida that I would like to sell you. Controlled studies of all these methods, show them to be no better than placebo (sham) treatments.[14]

Some health authorities suggest you should "practice" quitting, and that every quit attempt, even for a day, brings you closer to your goal.[14] This pat-on-the-back pseudo-psychotherapy is about as bad as advice can get. Well-trained psychologists associated with the Colgan Institute put it in the right perspective:

> *The strong emotional effects which condition the person to behave similarly in the future, occur not at the point of quitting but at the subsequent point of failure.*[15]

Consequently, a person who quits and fails is learning to fail to quit. Like the perennial dieter, for the perennial quitter, stopping smoking is easy. They've done it dozens of times. Don't fall into this trap.

Patch, Chew, and Spray

Numerous nicotine patches, gums, and nasal sprays are touted on television and the internet as sure-fire ways to stop smoking. These are simply alternative delivery systems for the same addictive drug, though without most of the cancer-causing effects of tobacco.

You should know that the tobacco conglomerates own and create most of these products. They don't give a damn what avenue they use to profit from the addictive power of nicotine, and they hold the world's biggest stores of the drug.

The patches are least effective because they allow only a continuous trickle of small amounts of nicotine into the bloodstream. Thus dopamine stimulation is minimal and unsatisfying. The gums, and especially the new oral sprays, give you a hit of nicotine up the olfactory epithelium, nearly as effective as a cigarette. At least they are better than smoking. Unlike second-hand smoke, nicotine gums and sprays also stay with the user and don't infect others around. They have a place as a *temporary* crutch to help you hobble towards quitting. Meanwhile, be warned, tobacco mavens are working their tails off to develop nicotine products even more addictive than tobacco.

Help Groups

The Government of Canada has a massive stop-smoking campaign, and thanks to new laws, many restaurants, bars, and other public places are now smoke-free. But their efforts have made hardly a dent in the number of individuals who smoke or the new generation of smokers training up to addiction. Their own figures show a less than 1% reduction in smokers from 2002 to 2003.[14]

Their e-mail program, their **On the Road To Quitting**, their **Quit 4 Life** program for young smokers, and the answers to their toll-free quit-smoking lines are a colossal waste of tax money. The programs are patronizing to the point of treating smokers like ignorant children, wordy to the point of boring the reader to sleep, and a perfect example of health authorities that display little knowledge of the nature of drug addiction and what is required to overcome it. No one with normal intelligence could find these programs effective.

The United States is no better. Each year the American Lung Association rates the country on the effectiveness of its government stop-smoking programs. For 2005, America got the following failing grades:

> Tobacco control .... D
>
> FDA tobacco regulation .... F
>
> Smoking cessation .... F[16]

So, you are mostly on your own. You have to quit yourself. The best help you can get is local, stop-smoking help groups. These volunteer organizations operate somewhat like Alcoholics Anonymous. The buddy or partner tactic is especially useful, in which two or more people combine to mentor each other out of smoking. They use the strongest incentives that the group can mutually agree upon, supported by a fund that all subscribe to. Money, fame, vacations, food, prizes, praise, even sexual favors, all work.

It's not easy to quit smoking, but it's the biggest health gift you can give yourself. I was a smoker until I was assigned to a terminal cancer ward as a part of my medical education. The abject horror of people dying in agony of lung cancer was enough to trigger the realization that it could also happen to me. Even so, it took me more than a year to quit.

Please, don't smoke! And don't let others puff their smoke about you. If you are a smoker now, you cannot be serious about health or longevity. It is well worth paying all you have to stay in a substance abuse clinic until you stop smoking. If you don't, then every other step you take to protect your health will come to naught.

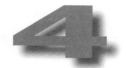

Overweight Causes Cancer

Impeccable research links smoking to 33%, and overweight to 25%, of all cancers.[1] Nevertheless, being fat is a far worse cancer risk than smoking, making this chapter the most important in the whole book. Why? Because most folk we survey still do not believe that body fat directly causes disease. They avoid smoking like the plague, but still treat big bellies as a bit of a joke.

Because of this general attitude, six people in every ten in America and Canada have allowed themselves to become grossly overweight, and the problem grows worse every decade. Unlike tobacco, which is now generally accepted as a potent carcinogen, the epidemic of obesity is clear evidence that most people still don't understand that *body fat is also a potent carcinogen*.

Folk tend to believe that being fat is more of a cosmetic problem. They seem unaware that the last 20 years of research have established beyond doubt that the adipose cell system is not merely a fat storage depot. It is also a collective endocrine organ which secretes a number of hormone-like substances into the bloodstream, such as **leptin**, which affect every other organ and system in your body, including your brain. When body fat gets above 18% in men and 22% in women, the influence of the adipose system becomes disproportionate, and the whole body begins to degenerate.

It is a huge indictment of American and Canadian medicine that treatment to reduce the serious illness of overweight is left largely to entrepreneurs, who fleece the public with cosmetic weight-loss programs so blatantly false they would make PT Barnum blush. Yet the science of becoming slim and staying that way for life is well established, ready to apply, and almost foolproof. I show you this science ahead. But first we will examine a few of the many links between body fat and cancer.

Fat Cancers

The American Cancer Society mounted one of the biggest studies ever of body fat and cancer, a massive 20-year examination of over one million Americans in 25 different states. Results showed unequivocally that overweight causes cancer. Men who are 40% or more overweight have higher rates of cancer of the prostate, colon, and rectum. Women who are more than 40% overweight have higher rates of cancer of the breast, uterus, ovaries, and gall bladder.[2]

A large body of research on women shows that you don't have to be obese. Increases in body fat mass and increases in waist-to-hip ratio with age, the typical "middle-age spread," progressively raise the risk of esophageal cancer, breast cancer, endometrial cancer, ovarian cancer, colon cancer, and uterine cancer.[3-9] Middle-aged spread is not a butt for humor, it is illness.

Body Fat Causes Breast Cancer

In a study representative of a mass of similar evidence, the International Agency for Research on Cancer analyzed the records of 11,663 women in a breast-cancer screening program. They found that the risk of breast cancer is significantly linked with overweight.[5] The fatter the woman, the higher the risk.

The most lethal form of breast cancer is inflammatory breast carcinoma. Only one in ten of its victims survive.[6] The University of Texas Anderson Cancer Center investigated all patients treated for this disease at the Center from 1985 to 1996. They concluded that overweight significantly increases risk. This increased risk was not influenced by menopausal status and was independent of other influences on breast cancer, including family history, smoking status, and alcohol use.[6] It's the body fat that does it.

Throat, Stomach, and Pancreatic Cancers

The National Cancer Institute recently reported rapid increases in esophageal cancer and gastric cancer. They also reported that the risk for these diseases rises in direct proportion to body mass index.[4] Fat bellies are walking billboards for the cancer budding silently inside.

The link between pancreatic cancer and overweight is also well defined. It works like this. Adult-onset diabetes is the end point of a decline in insulin metabolism. This decline is variously labeled insulin resistance, Syndrome X, or the CHAOS syndrome, depending on how far it has progressed. It affects almost everyone who becomes overweight. It is a strong risk factor for pancreatic cancer.[9] The National Cancer Institute measured that risk in an epidemiological study of people aged 30–79. They concluded that adult-onset diabetes increases your risk of pancreatic cancer by 50–60%.[10]

Pancreatic cancer is almost 100% fatal. It hardly seems fair that folk struggling with excess body fat plus diabetes should also risk the most deadly cancer, but that's the way the body crumbles. I will tell you ahead how to avoid it all.

Body Fat Causes Colon and Prostate Cancer

A representative study conducted by Kaiser Permanente, a medical insurance company, compared 1,983 patients with colon cancer with 2,400 matched controls, all aged 30–79 years. They concluded that obesity is strongly linked to increased risk of colon cancer.[11]

Another representative study, done at the University of Southern California School of Medicine, compared 483 cancer cases with 483 controls. They concluded that obesity, weight gain, and unstable adult weight (yo-yo dieting) are each *independent* risk factors for colorectal cancer.[12]

Overweight is also linked to prostate cancer. Using records from the Iowa 65+ Rural Health Study, researchers analyzed a database of 1,050 men aged 65–101 years over a 20-year period. This important long-term study showed that even moderate overweight increases the risk of prostate cancer. They also found that weight gain in later life is a potent risk factor for prostate cancer.[13] Don't let that middle-aged spread creep on.

Physiological Fattening

I could go on for the whole book documenting the links between body fat and particular cancers, but would rather turn to solutions. Here in a nutshell is the armor against body fat – for life. When it finally becomes adopted as the medical solution, remember you read it here first in 2006 and got a 10-year edge on the average game.

We know now that body fat increases with age, even if you don't change your eating habits, because of physiological changes in the human body. The three most important are:

1. Gradual decline of mitochondria, the energy-producing structures in our cells

2. Decline of the hormone cascade

3. Loss of insulin efficiency

There are many other changes that increase fat storage with age, but these three are the keys for most folk. They reduce the body's ability to convert food to energy, to maintain muscle, and to handle carbohydrates.[14] They are not addressed, nor even understood yet, by the diet industry.

Inactive Fattening

The fourth factor that fattens us up like Miss Piggy is inactivity. Modern life is labor saving to the point of killing us. Most folks choose not to move more than a few hundred meters unless they are carried by some sort of vehicle. From a genetic background of violent and extremely active evolution in order to survive, we the survivors now spend much of our lives immobile.

Unless you exercise regularly, the body has no way of maintaining an efficient system of using fat as fuel. An inactive person who becomes fat loses his or her ability to use the fat. It sits like sludge, clogging every part of the system: arteries, organs, and brain alike.

If you are fat and sedentary and don't believe us, then try this little test (with your physician's prior approval, of course). Weigh yourself. Now get on a treadmill or walk outside and continue walking until you are totally exhausted. Twenty miles or so should do it. Make sure to drink plenty of water to prevent dehydration. After the walk, don't eat anything. Simply go to bed.

A slim active person, whose fat fuel machinery is working well, will lose 2–3 pounds by the next morning and feel good. A fat, sedentary person will *gain weight* and will feel sick and exhausted to boot. When they weigh themselves next morning, despite having no food the night before, their weight will have *increased*. Their body not only defends every ounce of its fat, but also retains extra water to help it do the job. Don't fret, there is an easy way out of this dilemma.

Where's the Nutrition?

The fifth factor which predisposes us to overweight and cancer is abundance of the wrong food. With devilish cunning and monumental ignorance, food manufacturers extract the sights, tastes, and smells that tickle our inherited palates from their nutritious contexts in fruits and vegetables. Then they insert these hard-to-resist stimuli into the nutrition-less pap that lines supermarket shelves. So we still have the genetic urge to eat sweet and savory, sour and salt, but most of the foods we are offered to eat contain nothing but empty calories. I document the problems of modern food in detail in my new book, *Nutrition for Champions.*[14]

If these processed perversions of food form the bulk of your diet, the only way the body can survive is to learn to live off the food in its gut. Once it learns this trick, which takes a couple of years, you are condemned to eat pap every 3–4 hours or your blood sugar plummets. A healthy body eating real food lives from its structure and is not at all concerned if the gut isn't fed for even a whole day.

We use a simple test of body state that provides us with better data than any diet questionnaire. The subject presents for the test after fasting overnight. Water is permitted. We measure blood glucose level. The subject then walks briskly or runs for 10–15 miles (depending on fitness), with frequent water but nothing else. We measure blood glucose again at the end. If the body has a healthy diet and is living off its structure, blood glucose level shows no drop at all.

If the body has a pap diet, however, and depends on food in its gut for energy, blood glucose drops through the floor. Many of the pap-fed folk can't make five miles before hypoglycemia (low blood sugar) sets in. Don't worry. It's easy to change. I will give you the basics of bringing your body back to living off its structure.

Emotional Fattening

The final factor that fattens us up is emotional disturbance. Because food was hard to come by during our evolution, Nature programmed us with a strong drive to seek it and to eat gargantuan amounts whenever it was available. Areas in the hypothalamus of the brain connected with feelings of pleasure respond strongly to various tastes. Sweet and savory tastes, now usually buried in useless carbohydrates, are especially comforting to many women. Savory, sours, and fats that are equally buried in processed pap induce feelings of satisfaction in many men. These edibles only worsen the emotional problems, however, and make you progressively overweight to boot. There are far better ways to beat the blahs.

Winning the Body Fat Battle

To summarize the six main factors that fatten us up, they are:

1. Decline of mitochondria
2. Decline of the hormone cascade
3. Loss of insulin efficiency (rise of insulin resistance)
4. Sedentary lifestyle
5. Processed garbage foods
6. Emotional disorder

In this short book I can only sketch solutions, but sufficiently for you to get started. To get more details, read my books – *Nutrition for Champions,*[14] *The New Power Program*[15] and *Brain Power*[16] – or join the hundreds of folk who attend our summer seminars on beautiful Saltspring Island in British Columbia every year. Get details at www.colganinstitute.com.

Strategies to beat body fat have little to do with the temporary weight loss that makes dieting a multibillion dollar industry of repeat customers. They have nothing to do with the special meals, diet drinks, low-carb snacks, protein bars, or any of that useless commercial glop. ***To become slim and stay that way, you have to change the way that your body and mind react to food.***

Maintaining Mitochondria to Control Body Fat

Between ages 20 and 60 the capacity of the mitochondria, the energy-producing structures in your cells, declines by about 50%.[16] If the mitochondria cannot process the energy in the food you eat so as to release it, then your body has no alternative but to store it as fat. To prevent this problem, you have to maintain the mitochondrial energy system. The full program and scientific documentation for mitochondrial protection is given in my book, *Brain Power*.[16] Here I simply state the basics.

Most of the damage to mitochondria is caused by free radicals generated in the process of energy production. Usual antioxidants, such as vitamin C and vitamin E, have no protective effect because they cannot get into the cells in which the mitochondria reside. You have to use mitochondrial antioxidants, nutrients that are naturally metabolized inside the mitochondria. These nutrients are not yet well known, but they will be.

Table 4.1. Basic Nutrients Used by the Colgan Institute
to Protect Mitochondria

Nutrient	Daily Amount
R+ lipoic acid	200 – 800 mg
Acetyl-l-carnitine	500 – 2500 mg
L-carnosine	500 – 1000 mg
Idebenone	200 – 400 mg
N-acetyl cysteine	200 – 400 mg

© Colgan Institute 2006

Table 4.1 shows the basic nutrients used by the Colgan Institute to protect mitochondria. First, we use the mitochondrial antioxidant

R+ lipoic acid.   Second, we use the mitochondrial antioxidant **acetyl-l-carnitine**.   Third, we use the multifunction nutrient, ph buffer, and mitochondrial antioxidant, **L-carnosine**.   Fourth, we use the mitochondrial antioxidant **idebenone**, a derivative of coenzyme Q10.   Fifth, we use **n-acetyl cysteine**, the precursor of the endogenous mitochondrial antioxidant **glutathione**.

Many folk who attend our seminars have never heard of any of these nutrients in relation to losing body fat. Yet they are basic essentials to maintain your ability to convert food to energy. Without this ability, nothing else you do, even starvation, can have aught but a temporary effect.

Maintaining Hormones to Control Body Fat

Once you have protected energy production, the next step to control body fat is to protect your hormone cascade. Your hormone levels are primarily determined by the brain, with a cascade of its own hormones that occurs in both circadian (24-hour) and circannual (yearly) cycles. Decline of the hormone cascade, and consequent weight gain, insomnia, hot flashes, night sweats, depression, anxiety, memory loss, cognitive decline, and fatigue, is more obvious in women, who enter this degenerative state abruptly in perimenopause, between ages 35–45.[17] It also occurs in men, however, who enter what is called **viripause** more slowly, between ages 45 and 55.[17]

Again we can only sketch hormonal maintenance here, but sufficiently for you to understand the essential steps. Detailed analysis and full scientific documentation is given in my books, *Hormonal Health*[17] and *Brain Power,*[16] and in the *Colgan Institute Newsletter,* which is available at www.colganinstitute.com.

Hormone Replacement: Just the Facts

Hormone replacement is a hot topic because of the easily predicted increased cancer risk to women and subsequent warnings issued by the American Medical Association.[18] The increased risk is caused by horse estrogens and synthetic progestins used in the totally wrongheaded, complete waste of millions of your tax dollars, Women's Health Initiative studies. Ignorant press reports, or I should say misreports, have wrongly ascribed the same dangers to *all* estrogens and to natural progesterone.

Misled by the media, most folk we ask have many misconceptions about hormone replacement. And the usual medical use of HRT is, frankly, archaic. So we need to spell out the problem before we can show you the right way to overcome it.

You can't just throw in a glob of powerful, growth-stimulating, end-organ hormones, such as estrogen or progesterone, and expect all the cellular changes they induce to remain benign. Every living day, throughout your body, cells of every kind grow, divide, and replicate by the multi-billions, in response to thousands of competing signals from your hormones, your environment, every substance carried in your blood and lymph and concentrated in your organs, and everything you eat, drink, breath, sniff, or allow to get onto your skin. It is an exquisitely fine balance between all these chemical signals which determines whether resulting new cells are normal or abnormal. Balancing your hormones so that their signals remain benign is a continual chess game with Nature.

Putting in a glob of estrogen, progesterone, or testosterone, without first balancing the hormone cascade from the brain down, is like moving your chess pieces blindly, without paying heed to the positions of those of your opponent. Yet that is largely the state of

HRT today. There is an infinitely better and safer way.

Melatonin: The Master Control

Here I simply state the bare bones. To maintain your hormone cascade, first you have to maintain its timing mechanism. All our circadian rhythms, from the sleep/wake cycle to the release of luteinizing hormone, follicle-stimulating hormone, adrenocorticotropic hormone, and many others from the pituitary gland, the daily/monthly/annual rhythms of estrogen and testosterone, menstruation, reproduction, even libido, are timed and synchronized by the hormone **melatonin** from the pineal gland.

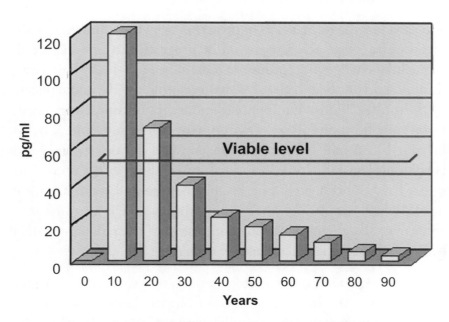

Figure 4.1. Decline of melatonin with age (Colgan Institute 2004).

Few of those who use this hormone as a common remedy for insomnia and jet lag realize that it is the master control. Without the steady influence of melatonin, which itself is controlled by daylight entering the eyes, the hormone cascade runs wild. The best example is night-shift workers, whose irregular daylight exposure disrupts their melatonin rhythm. Numerous studies show that this disruption increases their risk of cancer by about 300%. The cancer risk of the night shift is so well documented, we believe that those who work the wee small hours should be paid substantial danger money and well warned.

As shown in Figure 4.1, melatonin declines with age. A female over 30 and a male over 35 no longer make a sufficient amount to properly synchronize their hormones. The first step then to control body fat is to normalize hormone synchrony with melatonin supplements. Table 4.2 shows the amounts we use at the Colgan Institute.

Table 4.2. Melatonin Use at the Colgan Institute

Age	Males	Females
30 – 40 years	2.0 – 5.0 mg	0.25 – 3.0 mg
40 – 50 years	2.5 – 7.5 mg	1.0 – 4.0 mg
50 – 60 years	3.0 – 9.0 mg	2.0 – 5.0 mg
60 – 70 years	4.0 – 10.0 mg	2.5 – 6.0 mg
70+ years	5.0 – 12.0 mg	3.0 – 9.0 mg

© Colgan Institute 2006

Dopamine and Acetylcholine

The second step to hormonal maintenance is to maintain the neurotransmitters which control the flow of brain hormones from the pituitary gland, which in turn largely determine the levels of estrogen, testosterone, and many other hormones in your body. Estrogen and testosterone support your insulin system, partially determine how much muscle you carry and, in conjunction with the right food and exercise, how little body fat you carry.

It is crucial to note here that simply manipulating food and exercise, the usual approach to body fat, has *no* permanent effects. That's right, zero! All those high-fat, low-fat, high-protein, low-carb, food-combining, food-separating, Beverly Hills, Palm Beach, sugar-less, all-fruit, no fruit, Zone, zone-less, lose-all-the-weight-you-want diet books are worth naught but a good burning. For the right food and exercise to work, first you have to maintain your conversion of food to energy, your brain, and your hormone cascade.

The two most important neurotransmitters that we can influence, and that control pituitary output of hormones, are **dopamine** and **acetylcholine**. Both decline with age, beginning at about age 30. To maintain dopamine levels, we use **selegiline hydrochloride** in amounts of 1.0–6.0 mg per day depending on age. To maintain acetylcholine, we use its precursors **cytidine diphosphate choline**, 200–500 mg per day, and **phosphatidylserine**, 300–600 mg per day. The final basic item is **acetyl-l-carnitine**, the daily dose range of which we already specified for mitochondrial maintenance. Acetyl-l-carnitine does double duty by maintaining both mitochondria and acetylcholine.

Dehydroepiandrosterone (DHEA)

Downstream from the brain, it is also essential to maintain the level of **dehydroepiandrosterone (DHEA),** which is made from cholesterol in the adrenal glands. DHEA is the base material for manufacture of estrogen and testosterone. As shown in Figure 4.2, DHEA declines rapidly from age 25 onward. Without sufficient amounts of this hormone precursor, you cannot make your quota of end-organ hormones.

DHEA is also the body's most important repair signaling system. As DHEA declines, your body becomes less and less able to signal the brain and the immune system to send troops to clean up bits that have become diseased. Decline of DHEA is now thought to be a major cause of many degenerative diseases, including cancer.[19]

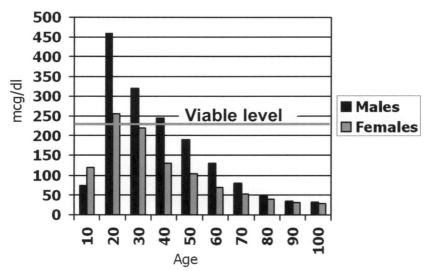

Figure 4.2. Decline of dehydroepiandrosterone (DHEA) with age.

DHEA is easily maintained by taking it in supplement form. At the Colgan Institute we use 10–50 mg per day, depending on six-month evaluations of the level of DHEA sulfate in an individual's blood. The level should remain within the accepted normal range for a person of 30, that is, 200–400 mg/dl. If DHEA becomes too high, we lower the dose accordingly, and vice versa.

In 1994, we fought alongside thousands of scientists to secure passage of Senator Orrin Hatch's *Dietary Supplementation and Health Education Act,* which gives Americans many important rights, including the right to buy DHEA over the counter. In some other countries, however, including Canada, Australia, and New Zealand, the health administrations are still controlled mostly by old physicians who did their medical training 50 years or more ago, when the health benefits of DHEA and many other chemicals were unknown. From their obsolete perspective, they have limited DHEA to prescription-only status, thus making it both difficult and expensive for the populations of those countries to obtain a most important, non-toxic, natural bulwark against disease. We have used DHEA in anti-aging programs for the past 30 years, with nothing but beneficial results. It is essential for many bodily functions, from direct prevention of cancer to control of body fat.

Hormone Replacement Therapy

After a certain age, in women from the onset of perimenopause between ages 35–45, in men from about age 45 on, end-organ hormones begin to decline, and body fat starts to creep on. Other degenerative changes loosely called "menopausal" occur about the same time. After 30 years of records of over 40,000 people who have taken programs with the Colgan Institute, we can state emphatically that hormone replacement therapy (HRT), correctly done, confers great benefits with little risk. These benefits accrue only if you have taken the steps outlined above to protect your mitochondria, your timing and repair signals, your brain, and your hormone cascade.

In this short account we will focus on women, whose problems with declining hormones are far worse than those of men. Optimal HRT for women concerns at least seven hormones: **melatonin**, **DHEA**, the three estrogens, (**estradiol**, **estriol**, and **estrone**), **progesterone**, and **testosterone**. Typical medical intervention attempts to replace only two, often using equine estrogen and synthetic progestins. This practice increases the patient's risk of reproductive system cancers, cardiovascular disease, gall bladder disease, and degeneration of the brain.[20-23] We strongly recommend against using these drugs, which do not match human hormones and cannot be controlled by the human system.

If you are going to replace one hormone, you have to replace all seven to have any hope of balancing the hormone cascade. You also have to use hormones that are biologically identical to those of human beings. Precise programs are way beyond the scope of this book, and I refer you to my book, *Hormonal Health,*[17] and to our website, www.colganinstitute.com, for details.

Maintaining Insulin Metabolism

Diabetes mellitus afflicts more than ten million Americans and about half a million Canadians. Probably twice those numbers are prediabetic and suffer progressive insulin resistance, that is, their insulin system is losing its ability to control sugar.

The majority of these people are overweight, but insulin resistance is more than just a cause of body fat. We know now that the loss of insulin efficiency happens gradually to almost everyone. It is a key factor linking five major degenerative diseases, now called the CHAOS complex: cerebrovascular disease, hypertension, adult-onset diabetes, osteoporosis, and stroke. Recently Alzheimer's disease, liver disease, and some forms of cancer have been added to the list.

Here we are concerned only with controlling body fat. Again I refer you to our other books for documentation of the medical literature. Here I simply state the solution boldly.

First, aim to eliminate sugar and highly processed carbohydrates from your diet. Second, take a complex of nutrients that increases insulin efficiency. These nutrients include:

DHEA: 10–50 mg per day (We have already specified this hormone precursor and daily dose under **Maintaining Hormones to Control Body Fat**, and we don't double up on the dose, but simply use the amounts there for double duty.)

Acetyl-l-carnitine: 500–2000 mg per day (We have already specified this nutrient and the daily dose under **Maintaining Mitochondria To Control Body Fat**, and we don't double up on the dose, but simply use the amounts specified there for double duty.)

Chromium picolinate: 1000–1500 micrograms per day

Niacin: 50–100 mg per day

Biotin: 5–15 mg per day

Manganese: 5–15 mg per day

Vanadium: 600–1200 micrograms per day

Methylhydroxychalcone polymer (MHCP): 10–20 mg per day

Docosohexaenoic acid (DHA): 1000–3000 mg per day

Eicosapentaenoic acid (EPA): 1000–3000 mg per day

Metformin

There is one other chemical I hesitate to mention because it is a man-made drug, and we are generally against the use of man-made drugs. With many people who have developed the pre-diabetic Syndrome X, however, it is an important adjunct to the above nutrients, both in controlling body fat and in inhibiting numerous other degenerative processes.

This important chemical is **metformin**, now widely prescribed for adult-onset diabetes. For the last decade, we have advised the physicians in many cases referred to us to utilize metformin in cases of Syndrome X, with outstanding results. Metformin does not suit everyone, however. It is very important that you *do not* use metformin unless you have the advice and consent of your personal physician to do so.

Syndrome X is characterized by all or most of the following conditions: high cholesterol (over 200 mg/dl), high triglycerides (over 100 mg/dl), elevated fasting blood sugar (over 105 mg/dl), overweight (over 27 BMI), and high blood pressure (over 130/85 mm Hg). It is a potent cause of cancer.

In conjunction with the other steps described to combat overweight, we have documented complete reversal of Syndrome X with use of a very moderate dose (500 mg per day) of metformin, without side-effects, as have many other researchers.[24] We were pleased to see in

August 2004 that metformin received a major review in the *Annals of Pharmacotherapy*, with the revolutionary conclusion that it be used for ***prevention*** of adult-onset diabetes.[25] Note well that the review does not say "treatment" but "prevention." As adult-onset diabetes is an inextricably linked part of the CHAOS complex of diseases, in effect this recommendation vindicates our decades-long advice that metformin is a most valuable aid in control of body fat and its links to many diseases, especially cancer.

I have to state again you ***must*** obtain the approval of your physician before using metformin, and all use must be regularly monitored by your physician. There are a number of other drugs and conditions such as pregnancy, liver inflammation, and infections that prohibit use of metformin. Overuse can also produce severe hypoglycemia and lactic acidosis which can prove fatal. Do not self-medicate with metformin under any circumstances. These cautions notwithstanding, we consider metformin to be an excellent preventative, without which many thousands of people would be condemned to insulin decline, overweight, and cancer.

You Can Beat Inactivity

Lack of exercise has become endemic in our labor-saved culture. And once the sedentary life has set in, exercise requires a huge effort and initially brings only pain and exhaustion. Nevertheless, regular exercise provides potent protection against cancer. One of the ways exercise protects you is by helping to control body fat.

But it has to be the right exercise that will support your body lifelong. Walking, jogging, aerobics classes, spinning, cycling, and all those treadmills, stair steppers, cross-country ski simulators, and elliptical gee-gaws are admirable in promoting cardiovascular fitness, but they are next to useless in controlling body fat.

Four main reasons. First, the usual 30–40 minute sessions of aerobic work 3–4 times per week use negligible body fat. We have documented the reasons in detail in previous books.[15, 26] Suffice to say here, that most overweight folk neglect the essential factor that enables use of significant body fat in aerobic exercise. Your stomach has to be empty when you do it. Otherwise, the body will use the food in the gut as energy and will leave your body fat practically untouched.

The second reason aerobic exercise is ineffective is that it takes 15–20 minutes of exercise for the body to make the hormone changes necessary to use any substantial amount of body fat as fuel. Even then, fat is released and used easily only if the hormonal signaling system is working properly. So at least half or more of every average aerobic session is burning predominantly sugar, not fat. And the rest of each session burns negligible body fat in folk who have lost the ability to properly signal the hormone cascade. That is the likely reason for anyone who eats properly and does regular aerobic exercise on an empty stomach, yet fails to lose much body fat.

The third reason for the failure of aerobic exercise to control body fat is that it does not maintain muscle. Muscle is the engine that uses body fat for fuel. You have to use a system of exercise that maintains muscle lifelong, such as the **Colgan Power Program.**

The final reason that aerobic exercise, or any other exercise for that matter, fails to control body fat is that the body will release the fat from adipose cells and use it for fuel effectively only if the ATP system, the hormone cascade system, and the insulin system are working properly. For many overweight people, it is mainly the failure of those systems that made them fat in the first place. So they have little chance of losing body fat (and beating cancer), except temporarily, until they have those systems repaired, as I have advised above.

For exercise, the members of the Colgan Institute all use the Colgan Power Program, a system designed to fit human anatomy and physiology, to maintain the structure and the muscles of the body lifelong. I cover the Power Program in detail in *The New Power Program*.[15] Here what you need to know to control body fat is do Power Program workouts at least three times per week.

Beating Emotional Body Fat

More than 25 million Americans and 2.6 million Canadians currently gobble gazillions of antidepressants and anti-anxiety medications in vain efforts to keep negative emotions under control. Short-term, these chemical straight-jackets relieve symptoms by numbing the brain, just like novocaine temporarily numbs the pain of an abscessed tooth. But pills and potions do nothing to root out the cause. Emotional disorder can never be cured by nutrients, medication, surgery, or any medical treatment, because it is rooted in your memory and triggered by your environment. It can be cured only by making changes to your mind.

To make these changes by yourself is difficult. To point the way, we want to share with you a brief look at the method we teach participants in Colgan Institute seminars on Saltspring Island in British Columbia, as well as seminars in the United States and New Zealand. It has enabled many folk to remove emotional stress from their lives. To do so is far more valuable to your health than any nutritional regime, any medication, any doctor, any other approach to life. We call it growing a **quiet mind**.

In all of us, the emotional residues of positive thoughts accumulate to form an underlying current of what the great Canadian physician Hans Selye termed **eu-stress**. While working with Dr. Selye in the 1970s, I learned how eu-stress cultivates a happy, confident, and resilient personality which promotes physical and mental health, strength and growth. I also learned how the emotional residues of negative thoughts, accumulate to form an underlying current of **dis-stress**. Dis-stress cultivates a sad, anxious, and fearful personality which promotes physical and mental illness, weakness, and premature aging.

Many of the emotional constructions humans attach to life events occur beneath the surface of consciousness. Thoughts invade the mind at such a rapid rate that we can give to each barely time to recognize its passing. Yet each thought excites emotional circuits in the brain that reverberate long after it is gone. These emotional residues often become permanent memories. A lifelong irrational fear of spiders, for example, can follow a single unpleasant experience of one crawling innocently into your ear.

The neural stimulation from such negative emotional memories affects hypothalamic-limbic-pituitary circuits in the midbrain, and disturbs the autonomic nervous system that controls all your housekeeping functions, from heartbeat, to appetite, to elimination. This disturbance can make you eat uncontrollably or not eat at all.

The Way of the Quiet Mind

For those who attend our seminars, we have developed the **Quiet Mind Program**. Quiet mind is a state in which the negative emotional baggage of your past can be viewed dispassionately for what it is — destructive emotional memories constructed by yourself. Just as you have placed each one, so the quiet mind enables you to remove it.

The source of the method is Zen. This system has been developed continuously for the last 2,500 years. The central practice of Zen, called **zazen**, involves sitting for a period each day in meditation. From our experience with thousands of athletes and folk seeking answers to aging and disease who come to the Colgan Institute, we have found that zazen is difficult for Westerners. Most of us are brought up to crave external stimulation. We are taught to revere busy-ness, and we live under the illusion that solutions to many problems can be acquired immediately, like instant mashed potato. To sit for a period each day, apparently doing nothing, seems appropriate only for the old and feeble. In 1996, we resolved to find an easier way.

Steps to a Quiet Mind

Over the last ten years, we have developed a method of contemplation more appropriate to Western culture. We teach people to meditate while busily in action, doing repetitive daily tasks, tasks that require little thought, such as tending a garden, jogging, and especially exercising in the Colgan Power Program.

In initial stages, with each repetition of the task, you are taught to focus on balance and breathing. Then, after some weeks of practice, you are taught to focus on greater and greater refinement of form and movement. Then, after some months of practice, you focus on less and less effort.

We use this method all the time at advanced levels of our Power Program. We teach athletes and others seeking extended healthy lives, to incorporate greater and greater **relaxation, coordination, rhythm,** and **fluidity** into all their movements. Gradually they become able to exert maximum force with very little effort or movement at all. Consciously doing the movement eventually becomes the movement doing itself.

Once you have reached this level of quiet mind, you can step back from your body and observe yourself. The unique causes of your emotional stress become more and more obvious, and easier and easier to eliminate.

You can then learn to do many life activities in quiet mind, which prevents new negative emotional memories from forming. The ultimate goal is to realize that every moment of life can be lived in this state, free from the damage of anxiety, anger, and fear, and certainly free from emotional eating and its attendant risk of cancer.

Lean for Life

It has been a long road in this, the most important chapter, to even sketch the basic strategies required for permanent control of body fat. But it is a road worth following. Together with not smoking, the simple strategy of remaining slim for life protects you from about *60% of all cancers*. Ahead we chip away at the remaining 40%.

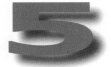

Our Food Is Degraded

Until the 1940s, farmers returned essential nutrients to the soil by mulching, manure, and crop rotation. These methods had worked successfully to maintain soil quality since agriculture began. But as agribusinesses grew, they saw no profit in Nature doing the work free of charge and claimed that expensive chemical technology could do a better job. So began the degradation of our food supply.

At the end of World War II, chemical conglomerates making nitrates and phosphates mainly for weapons were left with few buyers for their stockpiled mountains of products. They had to find new markets. Earlier experiments had shown that many plants will grow on a mixture of just three minerals: nitrogen (N), phosphorus (P), and potassium (K). With this knowledge, chemical manufacturers began making NPK fertilizers and selling them to farmers at attractive prices that made traditional soil enrichment methods uneconomic. By the 1960s, most farmers had become totally dependent on NPK products in order to make a living.

NPK fertilizers provide three of the main minerals essential for plant health. They grow fine-***looking*** crops with abundant yields. But your body is not a vegetable. It requires a much wider range of minerals. The US National Academy of Sciences states correctly that human bodies also need essential amounts of calcium, magnesium, selenium, chromium, iron, copper, iodine, molybdenum, zinc, cobalt, boron, and vanadium.[1]

These minerals used to be provided by traditional farming methods, which returned them to the soil in plant waste, and by plants grown especially for fertilization of fields allowed to lie fallow. From these practices, minerals enriched each succeeding crop. Today, fallow fields are history. Because of the widespread use of NPK fertilizers and intensified farming of crop after crop on the same ground, almost all soils in America have been depleted of numerous essential elements for human life since the 1970s.[2]

If soils are depleted of minerals, then crops are depleted, and so is everyone who eats them. That's you and me. Mineral depletion in the human diet increases the risk of numerous cancers. That's you and me again.[3] The latest survey shows that we get nowhere near the US Recommended Dietary Allowances of minerals from our food, even though most of us overeat. One in four Americans gets insufficient iron. Six in every 10 get insufficient calcium and magnesium. And three-quarters of us get insufficient zinc.[4]

Perils of Processing

The degraded foods produced on NPK fertilizers are further depleted of nutrients by mass-production methods of ripening, storing, drying, cooking, freezing, blanching, pasteurization, hydrogenation, ultra-filtration, and multiple other foibles of modern food processing.

The *Recommended Dietary Allowances* (RDA) handbook,[1] the official government analysis of the quality of American food supply has this to say about the depletion of nutrients:

> Vitamin E: *...the tocopherol content of foods varies greatly depending on processing, storage, and preparation procedures during which large losses may occur.* (p101)

> Vitamin C: *...may be considerably lower because of destruction by heat and oxygen.* (p117)

> Vitamin B6: *50–70 percent is lost in processing meats, and 50–90 percent is lost in milling cereals.* (p144)

> Folic acid: *...as much as 50 percent may be destroyed during household preparation, food processing and storage.* (p150)

> Magnesium: *...more than 80 percent is lost by removal of the germ and outer layers of cereal grains.* (p189)

Remember, these facts are not from scare-mongering media reports or tree-hugging hippies. They are direct quotes from scientific reports of the US National Academy of Sciences.

Where's the Beef?

Our meat supply is a similar horror story. In 1991, the Centers for Disease Control (CDC) in Atlanta released figures showing that approximately *half* of the 15 million pounds of antibiotics produced annually in America are used on livestock and poultry. We have bred animal grotesques for our meat, and we feed them on degraded slop. In order to keep them alive, over 90% of pigs and calves, 60% of cattle, and 95% of all poultry have antibiotics routinely added to their feed. Residues of these drugs contaminate most of the meat you eat.[5]

Where's the Fish?

Fish is little better. Wild fish now go mainly to gourmet restaurants, and unless you live at a fishing port, most of the fish you buy is farmed. Farmed salmon, other farmed fish, and shellfish have been indicted as strong risk factors for disease, including cancer.

In the *FDA Total Diet Study* covering 1991–1996, the Consumers Union published results of their investigation of the fish industry. They bought fish from the same places you buy it: supermarkets, grocery stores, and fish shops. Nearly 40% of this mainly farmed fish was beginning to spoil. Half the whitefish and 40% of the salmon were contaminated with polychlorinated biphenyls (PCBs). Over 90% of the swordfish were contaminated with mercury. The clams contained arsenic and lead. In the wild fish category, almost half of all the fish was contaminated with forms of bacteria usually found in animal feces.[7] Eat wild fish (except swordfish) or none at all.

Pesticides in Food

With traditional methods of soil enrichment, plants obtain the minerals and other substances from the soil that they require to make natural chemical compounds in their leaves, stems, and roots that discourage insects from eating them and microbes from destroying them. This system worked well for thousands of years. But plants grown in mineral-depleted soils no longer get enough of the nutrients required to produce their own insect and microbe-repellent compounds. Enter the chemical companies to manufacture synthetic chemical pesticides to protect the weakened crops and further poison our food.

It took a number of years, and overwhelming evidence that these pesticides were causing cancer and other diseases, before the government stepped in to begin to regulate the industry. In 1972, Congress passed a new act to protect America's food, water, and air and created the Environmental Protection Agency to enforce it. Enforcement has been a tad lax!

Under this milquetoast watchdog, staffed by a revolving door to the food industry, nearly 3 billion pounds of pesticides are spread in America every year. Currently used toxic pesticides include captan, alachlor, 1,3-dichloropropene, dinoseb, ethyl dibromide, lindane, pronamide, and trifluralin. We note these particular pesticides because they were cited as "***probable human carcinogens***" by the EPA's own special review process, way back in 1987.[6]

Because of ineffective enforcement and bowing to special interest lobbies, the EPA continues to allow use of more than 600 chemicals known to be harmful to human health. They form the basis of the 50,000 pesticide products in America today. If they are in our food, they are also in you and me.

The FDA conducts a yearly market basket program designed to monitor the levels of toxic chemicals in the US food supply. The latest figures up to 2000 showed *arsenic* in 24% of the foods analyzed. The highest concentration was found in seafood, followed by rice and rice cereals, mushrooms and poultry.[8] Arsenic is a proven carcinogen used in numerous pesticides and herbicides.

Studies done independently of the FDA show a worse picture. In 2000, a representative analysis found that contaminant exposures for the whole US population were high for arsenic, chlordane, DDT, dieldrin, dioxins, and polychlorinated biphenyls, all known carcinogens.[8]

The Wheat Debacle

The EPA's own studies of its lack of performance show clearly why cancer from pesticides is increasing. Take the example of chlorophenoxy herbicides. These chemical beasties are widely used both in cereal grain agriculture and in non-agricultural settings such as right-of-ways, lawns, parks, and golf courses. They are known carcinogens.[9]

Use of chlorophenoxy herbicides on wheat is a strong indictment of the EPA because wheat is used in so many thousands of food products. The states of Minnesota, North Dakota, South Dakota, and Montana grow the bulk of spring and durum wheat in the United States. More than 90% of this wheat is treated with chlorophenoxy herbicides. And cancer clusters around it.[9]

As wheat acreage in any area increases, so does cancer mortality. Not just one or two cancers either, but cancer of the esophagus, stomach, rectum, pancreas, larynx, prostate, kidney, urethra, brain, thyroid, bone, liver, cervix, ovary, and bladder.[10] That list covers most of our major body parts!

Many similar studies show these clear links between pesticides, herbicides, and cancer.   And even when the most dangerous chemicals are banned in the United States, you are far from safe. The banned chemicals are still manufactured and then sent to other countries where regulations are less strict.

Mexico is the worst because it ships most of its produce to the US, thereby sending the toxins back to our food supply.   A recent investigation shows that Mexico is the agricultural zone with the highest health damage to its population from pesticides.[11] Next time you see produce from Mexico, walk away from it – rapidly. And if a store does not know where its produce came from, or will not tell you, then walk away from it – permanently.

The solution is simple. ***Use only certified organic produce and meats and wild fish.*** Yes, it is more expensive, but not any way as expensive as disease. Every time you buy only certified organic produce for your family, pat yourself on the back for adopting a potent strategy to protect them against cancer.

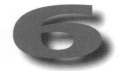

Refined Foods Promote Cancer

White bread doesn't cause cancer – directly. The problem of all refined flours is that refining destroys most of the nutrients required for their metabolism in the human body. White flour products, which include the bulk of breads, pasta, and baked goods, are so devoid of nutrients that even weevils cannot live on them for long.

At the Colgan Institute we introduced weevils into identical jars of white flour, enriched flour, whole-wheat flour, and mixed whole-grain flour, all kept in identical conditions of light, air, temperature, and humidity. By 60 days, most of the weevils and their progeny in the white and enriched flour jars had died. Those in the whole-wheat and mixed whole-grain jars thrived. If super-tough and adaptable animals like weevils cannot live on a food, neither can you.

Why did the "enriched" flour fail?   Surely it must be healthy with special vitamins added to it.   Wrong! Any college textbook of nutrition will tell you that human metabolism of carbohydrate requires at least seven vitamins and minerals: thiamin (B1), riboflavin (B2), niacin (B3), pantothenic acid (B5), pyridoxine (B6), phosphorus, and magnesium. If even one of these nutrients is not present in adequate amounts, your body cannot use the carbohydrate properly.

Almost the whole content of these seven nutrients is lost in processing of white flour. Usually only three vitamins – thiamin, niacin, and riboflavin – are added back to make enriched flour. These B-vitamins are put in to prevent vitamin-deficiency diseases that were common before 1940, but hardly exist today because of advances in medicine and public knowledge of nutrition. Enriched flour, however, remains in the food chain, an obsolete reminder of previous ignorance.

It is very difficult to add back all the required nutrients to refined flour because the synthetic vitamins and minerals used today differ chemically from the natural nutrients in grains. They often taste like vomit and affect baking characteristics, mouth feel, and a lot of the other complex characteristics of bread and baked goods.

With no commercial advantage for making enriched flour healthy, it hasn't changed in 65 years. Nutritionally, it is little different from white flour, as I have documented in other books.[1-3] Remember, nutrients always work in synergy.   If any one of the nutrients required for a specific task is missing, none of the others can work. It's simple biochemistry.[3]

White Flour IS Effective as Rat Poison

In order to use white or enriched-flour breads, pasta, and baked goods, your body has to rob itself, depriving nerves and muscle of pantothenic acid, depleting bones and heart of phosphorus and magnesium, and draining blood and brain of pyridoxine. In this way, high use of refined flour creates degenerative changes in the body that can lead easily to cancer.

If this sounds like exaggeration, consider studies done by nutrition expert Professor Roger Williams and his colleagues at the University of Texas. They fed one group of rats on enriched bread. They fed a second group on the same bread, plus a complete supply of vitamins and minerals. After three months, two-thirds of the enriched bread group had died, and the remainder had a variety of illnesses. The rats given the additional vitamins and minerals all thrived.[4]

White bread is even worse. In another study, a group of rats fed on regular commercial white bread were all dead within 60 days.[5] If white flour foods cannot support as tough and adaptable a creature as a rat, you have no chance of being healthy on it. You are simply laying the base for disease. Cancer is the grimmest set of degenerative diseases, always there, always waiting for any opportunity to proliferate.

Refined Flour Links to Cancer

Laboratory rats don't get to choose good food. But we do. Trouble is, most of us don't. Researchers examining data from the Iowa Women's Health Study found that many of the women used refined grains for more than 20% of their total energy intake and whole grains for only 1%. Results of the study showed a strong link between the refined grains and early death.[6]

Cancer of the gut is the likely executioner. Studies conducted in Switzerland show significant links between refined grain intake and colorectal cancer.[7] In the US, a study representative of the evidence was conducted by the Department of Nutrition at Harvard University. Results showed that high intake of refined carbohydrates also increases the risk of adult-onset diabetes.[8] This finding is important as there is firm evidence that hyperinsulinism (the beginnings of diabetes) plays a significant role in colorectal carcinogenesis.[9] Repeatedly throughout this book, we will see the link between refined starches and sugars, damage to your insulin metabolism, and cancer.

Use the Glycemic Index

Our simple cancer avoidance strategy for refined carbohydrates is the Glycemic Index. It refers to a food's ability to raise blood glucose levels. First developed by Dr. David Jenkins in 1971 to assist diabetics to stabilize their blood sugar, the Glycemic Index measures the magnitude of the blood sugar response to different foods. In most cases, the more the food is refined the worse it is. Pure glucose, one of the most refined carbohydrates, is taken as the standard, representing a 100% blood sugar spike.

To help you know what foods to avoid, Table 6.1 gives a short version of the Colgan Institute Glycemic Index. You can see where processed carbohydrates lie as compared to carbohydrates from fruits and vegetables. Processed carbohydrates are high-glycemic foods which spike blood sugar and insulin levels.

Table 6.1. Colgan Institute Glycemic Index*

High Glycemic Foods: 60–100%		Low Glycemic Foods: Below 60%	
Spike Blood Sugar & Insulin		Help Maintain Blood Sugar & Insulin Stability	
Avoid These Foods		**Eat These Foods**	
Breads	GI	**Breads**	GI
White wheat	72	Wholewheat pita	55
Cornmeal	68	Whole rye	52
		Pumpernickel	46-50
Baked Goods		**Baked Goods**	
Rice cake	94	Danish	59
Waffle	76	Bran muffin	59
Doughnut	76	Banana cake	55
Bagel	72	Sponge cake	48
Croissant	67		
Angel food cake	67		
Cereals		**Cereals**	
Puffed rice	90	Bran Chex	58
Rice Chex	89	Special K	54
Crispix	87	Oatmeal, old-fashioned slow-cooking	52
Corn Chex	83	All Bran	44
Cornflakes	77-83	Rice Bran	20
Rice Crispies	82		
Total	76		
Corn Bran	75		
Cheerios	74		
Puffed Wheat	74		
Shredded Wheat	69-77		
Grapenuts	67		
Instant Oatmeal	66		
Nutrigrain	66		
Pastas		**Pastas**	
White rice pasta	93	Spaghetti	56
Brown rice pasta	92	Linguine, durum	50
Gnocchi	68	Vermicelli	35
Macaroni	62		

Grains			Grains	
Instant rice	92		Brown rice	57
White rice	92		Buckwheat	54
Millet	75		Wholewheat	49
Cornmeal	68		Bulgur	48
Couscous	65		Whole rye	34
			Barley	23
Fruits			**Fruits**	
Dates	99		Papaya	58
Watermelon	72		Banana	46-54
Cantaloupe	65		Mango	55
Pineapple	65		Kiwi	49
Apricot, canned	64		Grapes	46
			Orange	40-48
			Peach	42-50
			Apple	33
			Pear	36
			Strawberry	40
			Plum	48
			Grapefruit	28
			Cherry	22
Vegetables			**Vegetables**	
Instant Potato	84		Sweet Potato	54
Baked Potato	83		Yams	51
Mashed Potato	75		Green Peas	48
Pumpkin	75		Tomatoes	38
Carrots	74		Squash	29
Beets	64		Cucumber	24
			Broccoli, cauliflower, cabbage, lettuce	Very low
			Peppers, onions, radishes	Very low
Legumes			**Legumes**	
None			Baked beans	48
			Pinto beans	42
			Butter beans	32

		Split peas	32
		Chickpeas	32
		Green beans	30
		Lentils	30
		Kidney beans	27
		Soy beans	24

Beverages		**Beverages**	
Canned juice nectars	72	Pineapple juice	46
Sodas	72	Grapefruit juice	48
Most fruit juices	60-70	Skim milk	32
		Milk	28
		Agave juice	15
		Tea	0
		Coffee	0
		Water	0

Snacks		**Snacks**	
Dates	99	Figs	59
Mini rice cakes	90	Popcorn	89
Popcorn	89	Oatmeal cookies	55
Graham crackers	74	Digestive cookies	54
Corn chips	73	Peanuts	18
Shortbread	64	Soybeans	18
Raisins	64		
Potato chips	62		

Candy		**Candy**	
Jelly beans	80	Plain vanilla ice cream	59
Skittles	70	Chocolate	50
Lifesavers	70	Peanut M & M's	35
Most hard candies	60-70		

Sugars		**Sugars**	
Glucose	100	Lactose	46
Honey	55-60	Fructose	40
Sucrose	65		

*Some lists use white bread as the 100% mark, which makes glucose 138–142%, depending on the standard you take. The pure glucose standard is more accurate because the blood sugar spike to white bread varies considerably depending on the flour used and numerous other factors. So stick to the glucose standard used with diabetics. © Colgan Institute 2002

Eating low-glycemic foods not only prevents adult-onset diabetes, but also helps prevent cancer. But you don't have to feel deprived. You can even eat the occasional banana cake or Danish, both of which just scrape into the low-glycemic range. If you keep your overall average food intake to about 50% on the Glycemic Index, you're doing fine to avoid cancer.

In agreement with the National Cancer Institute, we advise you to strike all white flour and enriched flour from your shopping list. Buy only whole grain, stone-ground, unbleached, and preferably certified organic flours. But read the labels carefully. Many breads and baked goods labeled "whole wheat" or "whole grain" are not.

Ingredients on food labels are listed in order of the amount contained in the food. When you read the ant-size letters of the ingredients list, whole grains may be the third or fourth ingredient, or not there at all. Mandatory food ingredients lists were developed in the United States as a health protective measure. Many countries don't have them. We're lucky to get the choice. As you will see, for most refined foods in the supermarket, folks would be a lot healthier ditching the contents and eating the package. Food packaging is not a known risk for cancer!

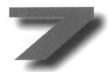

Toxic Water Everywhere

Every creature on earth is mostly water. Three-quarters of your brain is water. Your muscles are 70% water. Your blood is 82% water. Even your bones are one quarter water. Almost all your biochemistry can take place only in water. *The most important component of your body is plain H_2O.*

The quality of your muscles, bones, organs, and brain, their function, their resistance to injury and disease, and their longevity is absolutely dependent on the purity of the water that you drink. It has become a rare commodity.

Pure Well Water – Where?

Many people still have private well water. They commonly think this spring-fed water is cleaner than tap water because it does not go through any treatment system. It is not treated with chemicals such as aluminum and chlorine. But infectious and parasitic diseases are still the principal cause of death and illness throughout the world, primarily because of poor water quality. In 1997, diarrhea was ranked first in the world as a cause of illness and sixth as a cause of death.[1, 2] Diarrhea is caused mainly by contaminated water.

Like all commercial supplies, most well water is contaminated with man-made toxins. All drinking water, including well or spring water, is derived either from surface waters or groundwater. Water from either source is rarely pure. Increasing industrialization and urbanization which inevitably spawn toxic dump sites, together with intensified agriculture which contaminates water with fertilizers and pesticides, have decimated the pure water supply. In addition, we have all the microbes of civilization that breed happily in a water supply if it is not treated. If you drink well or spring water without having it tested for contaminants on a regular basis, you are playing Russian roulette.

Municipal Water Is Dirty Stuff

Modern treatment methods have reduced the possibility of bacterial or viral infections being transmitted in municipal drinking water. But most of the systems in America are now overwhelmed by demand. Waterborne microbial outbreaks have been reported in communities with even the best systems of water quality control. One of the notorious outbreaks happened in Wisconsin in 1993. Contaminated water supplies caused a widespread outbreak of gastrointestinal illness, mainly attributable to *Cryptosporidium*. This outbreak affected more than 400,000 people.[3] One big problem is that chlorination does not eliminate all waterborne disease.

Some pathogens are hard to kill. These include the Norwalk virus, hepatitis A, *Giardia* and *Cryptosporidium*.[4-6]

 Even Canada, with more water per acre than any other developed country and only a small population, cannot contain the infection problem.   Representative studies conducted in Quebec found that 14–40% of gastroenteritis was associated with tap water.[7,8] Remember, this water was meeting public health standards for water treatment and was considered by the authorities to be perfectly potable.

Health authorities are very aware of these problems, and there is endless debate in Canada and the United States about the urgent need for stricter water quality control and additional water treatment.[9] Though debate rages, little has been accomplished. If you drink tap water you continually risk disease.

To add to your health burden, by-products of chlorine themselves cause illness, including cancer. During the chlorination of drinking water, a complex mixture of by-products brews from chlorine and the organic and inorganic compounds present in raw water, including the carcinogens trihalomethanes and chloroform.[10] Gastrointestinal cancer and urinary tract cancer are strongly linked to chlorination.[11]

Researchers also estimate that 15% of bladder cancers in Ontario may be caused by drinking water containing relatively high levels of chlorination by-products. A report by the Center for Disease Control in Canada admits that the risk of bladder cancer from drinking water is an important public health problem.[12]

Arsenic is another major water contaminant widespread in the water supply. This is a problem for both untreated water and municipal water.   Arsenic is very difficult to eliminate from water using conventional methods.   Arsenic in drinking water is a recognized cause of cancer of the skin, lung, and bladder.[13, 14]

The Quest for Clean Water

So what are the alternatives? The bottled water industry is booming. But many of these products are simply tap water passed through "conditioning filters" such as charcoal, which eliminate some of the chlorine and unpleasant tastes and odors. These filters do not remove the toxins.

What about "spring" water? Brands labeled "Spring Water" legally have to be from a spring unless the words are a brand name or part of a brand name. Then they are just tap water. Spring water, however, is just untreated groundwater. Whatever goes into the surrounding ground ends up in the spring water. Today, spring water is no more pure than well water.

Springs also contain all kinds of organic matter and often some very toxic minerals. A test of a well-known bottled spring water imported from West Germany showed excessive levels of selenium and cobalt, and a level of arsenic that exceeded the EPA standards by 6000%.[15] The purity of bottled water is often a figment of greedy imaginations.

Distill Your Water

The only reliable bottled water is distilled water. Virtually everything is removed by steam distillation, leaving almost pure H_2O. And because distilled water is often used for medical purposes, the companies that produce it have more rigorous standards.

Bottled distilled water, however, is very costly. An excellent alternative and a potent anti-cancer strategy is to put in your own purification system to clean your tap or well water for drinking and cooking. From our writings on water over the last two decades and the work of many other scientists, a lot of new houses are now having whole-house distillation systems installed that purify all water entering the house. Now that's clean!

For most people a whole-house system is not a practical solution. But there are many good systems available that install in or near your kitchen that provide plenty of clean water for your family. Simple charcoal filters will not do. These do not remove the majority of contaminants. A good reverse osmosis unit that is serviced regularly will bring your water down to about 30 parts per million of dissolved solids. This is reasonable when you consider that most tap water is 300–600 parts per million of dissolved solids.

The best system, however, is a home distiller which also incorporates a solvent vent that vents outside the house. There are excellent products available that are no more trouble to service than your dishwasher. Some of the best are available through Pure Water Inc (www.purewaterinc.com). A good distiller will clean your water so that it is between 0–15 parts per million of dissolved solids. At least as clean as a whistle.

Some folks object to this purity, complaining that the very emptiness of distilled water causes it to leach minerals from the body. Anyone with a basic understanding of biochemistry knows this is impossible. As soon as you drink it, water becomes a soupy mixture with all the contents of your gut. On absorption through the intestinal wall, the mixture immediately blends with your body fluids and becomes part of you. There is no physiological way it can suck minerals out.

Other folk claim that you are missing your minerals by not getting them from your water. Certainly some studies have shown that "hard" water, that is, water with a high level of minerals, especially calcium and magnesium, is heart protective. But it is not the drinking water that does the trick. Most of the minerals are concentrated in the food you eat that is grown on these mineral-enriched soils. If we were to rely on the miniscule amount of minerals in water for our minerals, we would all be in a bad way.

It is the fruits, vegetables, and grains that take up the minerals and concentrate them sufficiently to provide our mineral requirements. Dr. Eric Underwood, a world expert on minerals in food, states it plainly,

> *Plant materials provide the main source of minerals to animals and to most members of the human race.*[16]

Drink and cook with water as pure H_2O and put another tick on your cancer prevention program.

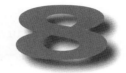

Cancer At Home And Work

Your home may be hazardous to your health. Tobacco smoke is an obvious hazard. Toxic gases also leak silently, undetected, from plywood, particle board, carpets, drapes, furniture, and plastics. Many of these gases are carcinogenic.

Take formaldehyde as an example. New materials can exude formaldehyde gas for up to eight years.[1] Inhaled formaldehyde readily induces nasal squamous cell carcinoma. As a health risk, exposure to even six parts per million in air, especially in combination with sinus problems or chemical sensitivity, quadruples the risk of lung cancer.[2] If you have just moved into a new home or have new carpets, etc., keep the air in the house circulating with outside air. If you are building a new home, the best quality plywood, insulation, and wall board are now formaldehyde free.[3] Insist on them.

Radon Gas

Another carcinogenic hazard in your home is radon gas. Radium is a naturally-occurring mineral component of soil and rock. Radon gas is its decay product. The gas seeps through the ground and through unsealed foundations and crawl spaces, and accumulates in homes. Unsealed basements and crawl spaces are left that way to cut costs in many new houses. They provide an open channel for radon to seep up and accumulate in sealed living spaces where it can't get out. Indoor radon is a recognized risk for lung cancer.[4]

The US Environmental Protection Agency now recommends that all dwellings be tested for radon. Homes with radon levels exceeding 148 Bq/m³ should be promptly treated to remove the gas.[5] But most people don't bother to have the tests done because you can't see, smell, or taste radon. Don't be one of them.

If you do find hazardous radon levels, single treatments and open windows are not enough. Radon will seep continually from the soil beneath the house. The solution, however, is simple. Seal all basements and crawlspaces from the ground with a plastic membrane and ventilate them.

To keep this risk in context, in terms of an overall cancer prevention strategy, it is important to recognize that a miniscule reduction of 0.05% in the number of people smoking would prevent as many deaths from lung cancer as are caused by all the radon exposure in America.[5] If you seal your home against radon, but then allow anyone to smoke in it, you need not have bothered.

Pesticides at Home

A more serious cancer risk in your home is exposure to pesticides, insecticides, and herbicides. These include all the sprays for fleas, ants, flies, wasps, and termites; flea collars on pets; pest-strips; herbicides to control weeds in the garden or orchard; and pesticides to control bugs on outside vegetation. Children are especially vulnerable to this type of exposure. If it says safe on the label, they are lying through their teeth! If chemicals are toxic enough to kill bugs and weeds, they are also toxic to you.

Cancers in children linked to pesticide use in the home include leukemia, neuroblastoma, Wilms' tumor, soft-tissue sarcoma, Ewing's sarcoma, non-Hodgkin's lymphoma, and cancers of the brain, colorectum, and testes.[6-8] Every single one of these cancers can be prevented by not bringing these chemicals into your home.

Your dog is not only a watchdog against intruders, but also a potent watchdog against cancer. Canine malignant lymphoma and sinonasal cancers in dogs are linked to chemical exposure in the home.[9, 10] The list includes all the chemicals above, plus the carcinogenic by-products of burning fossil fuels such as coal and kerosene. Like the canary in the coal mine, your dog's superb senses are more subject to damage than yours. If your dog (or cat) develops cancer, look carefully for hazardous chemicals you use in and around your house. Eliminate them.

Cancer at Work

Many of the carcinogens used in homes are also a problem in the workplace. Formaldehyde, for example, is used in the garment industry and in the plywood and particle board industries. It is also used in the manufacture of adhesives, detergents, dyes, fertilizers, insecticides, leathers, paints, paper, and plastics. If you work in these industries, you are at risk of cancer, no matter what the plant safety inspector says.[11]

Any industry that exposes you to inhaled chemicals or any type of dust is a cancer risk industry. The same goes for work on the land. If you are involved in non-organic farming, then be aware of the risk to yourself, your family, and your neighbors from uncontrolled or incorrectly used fertilizers, pesticides, and herbicides.[12] It bears repeating that any chemical that kills plants or bugs can kill you.

Your best prevention is awareness and care. There is a rule in most laboratories, "If you can't eat it, don't touch, taste, or inhale it, or allow it to get onto your skin." It's a good cancer prevention strategy to adopt at home and work, to protect you and your family from the thousands of toxic chemicals that pervade our environment every day.

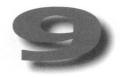

Ultra-Violet Causes Cancer

Solar radiation is the most important environmental stress agent for human skin. It causes premature skin aging and multiple forms of skin damage. Over the last decade a mountain of evidence confirms that exposure to ultraviolet light causes skin cancer.[1]

In 2000, an estimated one million Americans were diagnosed with skin cancer. This accounted for an amazing 50% of all new cancers.[1] Skin cancer is so common that, except for melanomas, it is not even included in the cancer statistics. Worldwide, the incidence of skin cancer is increasing more rapidly than any other malignancy. Despite intensive educational efforts by the medical community, the public has not learned.

Skin cancer comes in three main forms – basal cell carcinoma, squamous cell carcinoma, and melanoma. These cancers occur most frequently on the sun-exposed areas of the head and neck. About

90% of non-melanoma skin cancers, and much of the incidence of melanoma, are caused by simple exposure to the sun.[1] So more than 90% of skin cancers are preventable because sun exposure is a lifestyle choice.

Recent evidence indicates that regular use of sunscreen (SPF 15 or higher), wearing protective clothing and wide-brimmed hats, and avoiding sun exposure when the ultraviolet rays are strongest (between 11 am and 3 pm) dramatically reduces the risk of skin cancer.[2]

Tanning Beds

A big hat will not protect you from tanning in a UV bed or stall. A concerned parent asked me, "Surely they wouldn't allow tanning beds if they caused cancer?" My reply was, "*They* still allow tobacco, madam."

Once and for all, the evidence is overwhelming that tanning beds cause skin cancer — no matter what the marketers say about their particular lamps. The US National Cancer Institute, the American Cancer Society, the National Institutes of Health, the British Institute of Cancer Research, the Canadian Cancer Society, and the World Health Organization all issue strong warnings that tanning beds, booths, sunlamps, and any other weird UV devices ***increase your risk of skin cancer***.

The largest study on tanning bed use was completed in Sweden in 2003 and published in the *American Journal of the National Cancer Institute*. It followed 106,000 women using a huge variety of tanning beds, booths, and other devices. Results were clear. Women who used any of the methods more than once per month increased their risk of malignant melanoma by 40–130%.[3] Melanoma is the deadly one. Don't use tanning beds. If you want a tan, get it from a bottle. It's a simple lifestyle choice that prevents a lot of cancers.

Of the three different forms of skin cancer, melanoma accounts for 75% of all deaths. It may start as only a tiny new mole or pimple that will not heal, but once its tentacles have spread around the body, the chance of a cure is remote.[2-5] Deaths from melanoma have risen rapidly in the past decade. In Britain, for example, not famed for sunny skies, melanoma deaths have risen by one-third in the last decade.[4] A new mole, a mole that changes, or a mole or pimple with irregular colored edges should send you to the doctor for its prompt removal. Getting the melanoma before it has spread is *the* way to beat this terrible disease.[3]

Protect Your Children

Adolescence is the highest risk period for development of melanoma and other skin cancers later in life. Like many other cancers, seeds of skin cancer are often planted early and usually germinate into full-blown disease after many years. If you suffered even a single bad sunburn (that raised blisters), be alert for any unusual lumps, bumps, or other changes in your skin as you age, and get them removed promptly.

Representative studies show that less than one-third of American teenagers protect themselves from the sun.[6] Similar research in Australia, the worst country in the world for melanoma, shows that teens now protect themselves from the sun a whole lot more than they used to. Since melanoma deaths sky-rocketed in Australia and New Zealand during the last decade, coincident with the growth of the hole in the ozone layer over those countries, two–thirds of their teens no longer go out to the beach to tan.[7]

What about the commonest cancers of all, basal cell and squamous cell carcinomas of the skin? Make no mistake, even non-melanoma skin cancer can be is deadly. We are currently observing the efforts of a whole team of specialists trying to prevent the death of a woman with squamous cell carcinoma developed from tanning. It's difficult, but they might just win.

All this caution doesn't mean that you can't enjoy the summer beach or the mountaintops. Simply use plenty of waterproof sunscreen and a big umbrella on the beach. Don't let even a pinky get sunburned.

10

Alcohol and Cancer

More than 100 studies piled on my desk show a clear association between alcohol and cancer. The main demons are cancer of the oral cavity, the pharynx, the larynx, the esophagus, and especially the liver.[1] In their prestigious report, *Diet, Nutrition and Cancer*, the US National Research Council also specifically linked excessive beer drinking with colorectal cancer.[2]

Nevertheless, the link between alcohol and cancer is more subtle than it is with smoking. Alcohol is far and away the favorite drug of Western Society. Yet, despite the huge amounts consumed every day, it causes cancer in less than 1% of drinkers. That's tiny compared with the 33% of smokers who get cancer from tobacco.

Alcohol is not directly causative either. Experimental studies in animals show that **ethanol** in alcohol is not a carcinogen by itself, but under certain conditions can become a co-carcinogen, in combination with other risk factors. In the liver, alcohol is more a tumor promoter than a direct cause.[3]

We know that the metabolism of ethanol leads to the generation of **acetaldehyde** and other free radicals. These highly reactive toxic compounds bind rapidly to cell constituents and possibly to DNA. Acetaldehyde interferes with your DNA repair mechanisms. It also traps glutathione, an important antioxidant in detoxification, and contributes to breaks in chromosomes. It's a gremlin you can well do without.

An enzyme in your body called **aldehyde dehydrogenase-2** normally eliminates most of the acetaldehyde produced during alcohol metabolism. In heavy drinkers, however, the activity of this enzyme is dramatically reduced, thereby increasing their risk of cancer.[4]

How Much Alcohol?

How much alcohol does it take to increase your risk of cancer? No one knows. Good estimates indicate that one American in every five drinks too much for good health.[5] That's over fifty million of us! Confirmed alcoholics number about 17 million. With that level of consumption, alcohol makes a hefty contribution to the cancer load.

It's a fair bet that the level of alcohol intake that causes other degenerative disease also increases cancer risk. A survey of all relevant studies by the Colgan Institute agrees with the conclusion reached by a similar survey done at Harvard Medical School. More than ***one-and-a-half ounces*** of alcohol per day results in slow degeneration of the liver.[6] Your liver is the main organ of detoxification of the body. Anything that reduces its function increases your risk of a wide variety of disorders.

A regular size drink contains approximately half an ounce of alcohol. So the upper limit, if you want to prevent cancer, seems to be three beers, *or* three glasses of wine, *or* three singles of liquor.

Not Just the Alcohol

It's not just the alcohol. Over 1,000 chemicals are added to alcoholic beverages, and up to the present, the liquor industry has successfully resisted all attempts to make them tell the public what these chemicals are. It is a sad commentary on American health authorities that they insist on non-carcinogenic cookies being labeled down to the last innocuous ingredient, while carcinogenic alcohol products continue to feed us hundreds of toxins blind.

One very important criterion is product quality. At the Colgan Institute, for research purposes, we managed to obtain a full listing of ingredients of some brands of red wine, under the strict stipulation that we would not publish this information. What we can tell you is that cheap plonk wine contains way more toxins than high quality wine. Saving a few dollars on that bottle of wine for dinner is not a smart form of economy.

What's Your Tipple?

Cancer risk may also depend on the form of your favorite drink. A representative recent study conducted in Denmark concludes that a moderate intake of wine does not increase the risk of upper digestive tract cancer, whereas a moderate intake of beer or spirits increases the risk considerably.[7] In your quest to prevent cancer, you can still enjoy a couple of glasses of alcoholic drinks per day, but make them first-class wine. Go for quality over quantity every time.

If you do drink, then protect your liver with **silymarin**. This simple herbal has garnered great praise from researchers as armor for the liver against multiple toxins from hepatitis to pesticides to alcohol and other known carcinogens.[8]

11

Infections Cause Cancer

More good news. When I wrote my first book on prevention of cancer in 1990, we knew that some chronic infections caused about 7% of all cancers in America and Canada. But we were not sure which ones were the worst culprits and didn't really know what to do to prevent them.[1] Now we know a lot more, and can do a lot more.

There are three main mechanisms by which infections cause cancer: direct effects of some viruses; chronic inflammation caused by a long-term infection, such as a stomach ulcer caused by the bacterium *Helicobactor pylori*; and viral agents such as HIV which weaken immunity. You cut all the risks from these infections by at least 60% right away when you practice good nutrition, good hygiene, and safe sex,[2] and also maintain strong immunity as detailed in Chapter 19 ahead.

The known infections that can cause cancer are shown in Table 11.1. I say "can cause cancer" because most cases of these diseases don't. In some parts of the world they account for over 20% of all cancers, but in the US, Canada and most developed countries, only 5–8%. That's more than enough, seeing that they are almost all preventable.

Table 11.1. Infections That Can Cause Cancer

Infection	Main Form of Cancer
Schistosomes	Bladder
Liver flukes	Bile duct, liver
Helicobactor pylori	Stomach
Hepatitis B virus	Liver
Hepatitis C virus	Liver
Papilloma virus	Cervix, anus, penis, oral
Herpes virus Type 8	Kaposi's sarcoma
HIV-1 Lymphoma	Kaposi's sarcoma
T-cell lymphotrophic virus	Leukemia
Epstein-Barr virus	Hodgkin's, Burkitt's

© Colgan Institute 2006

Schistosomes are microscopic trematode worms that take up residence in the bladder. People in developed countries get infected all the time by drinking supposedly pure water from lakes and streams. They especially get infected from drinking water in glamorous tourist destinations in not-quite-developed countries, such as Mexico, and all third-world countries. Easy to prevent. Don't drink the water. A few years ago I spent six weeks lecturing at universities in China and drank bottled, very weak, Chinese beer for breakfast, lunch, and dinner. It was the only safe beverage available. Schistosome infections are now easily identified and very treatable with drugs, even after long infection and development of serious bladder disease.[3]

Liver flukes are two types of little parasite that invade the bile duct. They are unknowingly acquired from eating raw fish, especially fresh-water fish, especially overseas. Developing countries – don't even go there – liver flukes are rampant. Liver disease from liver flukes has to be surgically removed.[4] Nasty. Prevention is obvious, simple, and painless.

Helicobactor pylori is a bacterium, so named because it looks like the blades of a microscopic helicopter. About half of US adults over 60 and about 20% of younger folk tested show *H. pylori*. We know now it is responsible for most stomach ulcers and most stomach cancers,[5] although it doesn't seem to bother the majority of its hosts.

H. pylori was discovered in 1982 by Australian researchers Barry Marshall and Robin Warren, who then spent the next decade defending their find. It was not generally accepted as the main cause of stomach ulcers until 1994. Since then, most cases have been curable with antibiotics, and the infection doesn't stay around long enough to cause cancer. Good to record that the stomach cancer rate has plummeted since 1995.[6]

More good news. **Hepatitis B**, which causes liver cancer, is now eminently preventable (along with hepatitis A) by the Twinrix vaccine. Yeeeeeess… I've heard all the arguments for and against vaccines for more than 30 years now. But I worked under Jonas Salk for a while and saw polio disappear with his magic science. I also saw smallpox disappear. That's what science is all about. All

Colgan Institute folk have had the Twinrix shots. It's just common sense.

Just as an extra about vaccines, I'm also hugely in favor of the pneumococcus vaccine and the annual 'flu shot. Do not suffer these ancient diseases. You don't have to compromise your immunity with them. There's more than enough cancer and other diseases about that your defenses have to take care of.

Hepatitis C, which also causes liver cancer, is not conquered yet. It was only discovered 16 years ago, but vaccines first went on trial in 2001. Now in May 2006, the big trial and push for FDA approval have just begun at St. Louis University School of Medicine. We are hoping it will pass muster and add one more piece to our armor against cancer.

Cancer specialists first suspected the link between **human papilloma virus (HPV)** and cervical cancer in the 1970s. By my entry onto the cancer scene in the 1980s, scientists accepted that almost all cases of cervical cancer are caused by one or another of the multiple forms of this pesky little invader. It is spread by sexual contact, which is why it also causes oral and anal cancer. Two virulent forms that cause these cancers, HPV 16 and HPV 18, were isolated from cervical cancer biopsies in 1983 and 1984. These were called "High-risk HPV."[8] Cervical cancers are the second most prevalent form of cancer in women.

Contrary to scary stories, most HPV forms that are isolated from genital warts are not High-risk HPV and seldom develop into cancer.[8] They do cause other disease, however. Casual sex and sex with sex trade workers is a huge source of all sorts of gremlins. On a holiday in Mexico, one of my resourceful colleagues was approached by a prostitute who was operating in the 5-star resort and was feeling sick. After examining her, and with the hotel's blessing, he rushed off to the local university lab he had been visiting and cultured 39 separate infections from her vaginal secretions.

Contrary to common advice, use of condoms does not offer much protection against HPV because virus-infected cells lurk on the skin and mucous membranes all around the outside of the genitalia. Prevention by condom is almost impossible if you have multiple sex partners. An estimated 20 million Americans are now infected.[8] Even if you do form a monogamous relationship, get tested – both of you.

There is some good news. Simple microbicides in cream or gel form are almost on the market. Used in conjunction with a condom or on a special diaphragm, they prevent the transmission of papilloma virus. Buffergel, manufactured by ReProtect LLC in Baltimore, is in Phase 3 clinical trials. It not only stops papilloma virus, but also herpes, chlamydia, and most HIV. It doesn't work against gonorrhea.[9] Not far behind in clinical trials is PRO 2000, an antimicrobial that blocks all the above, plus gonorrhea and syphilis as well.[9] The two together are a formidable weapon against STDs and their cancer-causing potential.

By the 1990s, the race was on to find a vaccine against HPV. In the last two years, the vaccine Gardasil, developed by Merck, passed all the necessary clinical trials. It effectively blocks the high-risk HPV and also two forms of the virus that cause genital warts. A second vaccine, Cervarix, developed by GlaxoSmithKline, is also on the way to approval.[10] On Thursday, 18 May 2006, a federal advisory panel unanimously recommended that the FDA approve Gardasil for women and girls from age 12 up. As I write this, the Center for Disease Control is due to meet on 29 June 2006 to decide how Gardasil will be released.[11] Excellent news.

Herpes virus Type 8 and HIV are also sexually transmitted diseases that cause cancer. T-cell lymphotrophic virus is endemic among the very poor and some migrant populations coming to the United States, and among drug users who inject and their sexual partners. I covered prevention of these nasties in the STD bit above. No need to labor it further.

Popularly dubbed "the kissing disease," Epstein-Barr virus is the subject of a lot of public hype and flapdoodle. Here are the facts. It's not a rare and mysterious infection. It is as common as the common cold. Famous British surgeon Denis Burkitt first suspected its existence in 1961 as the cause of the cancer named after him, Burkitt's lymphoma. Two researchers named Michael Epstein and Yvonne Barr led the team that isolated the virus in 1964, for which they got their 15 minutes of fame. It turned out to be a common herpes virus, HV-Type 4.[12]

Epstein-Barr virus is spread through mixing your saliva with that of an infected person, whereupon it promptly takes up residence in your salivary glands. Most Americans are infected during childhood, usually by loving kisses from their father, mother, or grandparents. Over 80% of Americans then carry Epstein-Barr for the rest of their lives and pass it on to their own children. In the vast majority of cases, it never bothers us, being kept in check nicely by our immune systems.

Only when immunity fails does Epstein-Barr raise its ugly little head, popping out as mononucleosis, which used to be called glandular fever. That's why mono is common in transplant patients whose immunity has to be kept suppressed. It's rampant in folk with HIV, which directly compromises immunity. It's also common in elite athletes, especially when they overtrain to be ready for top competitions such as the Olympic trials and shoot their immunity (and their chances) in the foot. In rare cases, long-term active Epstein-Barr eventually causes cancer.[12]

Prevention of mono and other Epstein-Barr diseases is a balancing act. Keep your immunity strong with the strategies in Chapter 19 and you should have no trouble. But neglect your nutrition or exercise, or chronically overwork, or chronically overtrain, and it will likely sock you good.

I hope that this chapter has given you the armor to resist the cancers known to be caused by infections. Most are not difficult to avoid, but if you do get symptoms of any of the infections above, have it treated promptly. Curing active infections is the key to prevent them triggering cancer.

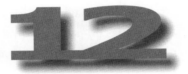

Low-Fat Diet Prevents Cancer

The American diet is still 34–41% fat. Yet US health authorities repeatedly recommend that everyone keep fat intake below 30% of total calories. Dietary decrees are easy to say. But, because the same health authorities have permitted the degradation of our food supply, they have made the task of eating a low-fat diet about as easy as opening a can of beans — with your nose.

Many folk who come to the Colgan Institute firmly believe they follow a low-fat diet. But when we analyze what they actually eat, it often turns out to be drowning in grease. A bran muffin, for example, can contain more lard than a plate of french fries. Low fat turkey roll can be higher in fat than ice-cream. And dry crackers are usually dripping with dripping.

The *New York Times* did a poll of the diets of 1,870 people in 1999. Over half the respondents claimed they had cut right down on fats and cholesterol. Yet their responses to other questions showed regular meals of red meats, whole eggs, fast foods, ice cream, and a ton of foods with hidden saturated and trans fats. On 25 May 2006, in the same newspaper, market researcher Leo Shapiro reviewed how little diets had changed since.[1] His conclusion:

> *Almost all people just trade one fat for another. If they don't have the burger, they are going to have the fries.*

Many folk have the best intentions to cut down on fat, but lack the knowledge to do it. To prevent cancer you need this knowledge, because you don't have to be fat in order to risk cancer. You just have to eat the wrong fat.

Fat Causes Colon and Breast Cancers

We first learned that dietary fats cause cancer from animal experiments. A representative study from the medical journal *Nutrition and Cancer* compared the effects of various types of fat on cell proliferation in the colon. Cell proliferation is the prelude to polyps, which often develop into colorectal cancer. Four groups of rats were each fed a diet containing 45% of total calories from fat, just a tad above what most Americans eat. The high fat diets used corn oil, butter, beef tallow, or fish oil. A control group was fed a low-fat diet containing only 15% of total calories from fat. Results showed that the high fish oil diet and the very low fat diet were protective. The high corn oil, beef tallow, and butter diets all caused growth of precancerous cells in the colon.[2]

Another representative study from the same journal induced mammary gland tumors in female rats, then placed them on a high corn oil or low corn oil diet for 25 weeks. The high-fat group developed more tumors and had a higher incidence of cancerous tumors. The authors concluded that high-fat diets increase the incidence, invasiveness, and growth of mammary gland carcinomas.[3]

The National Research Council of the US National Academy of Sciences has published similar strong evidence linking dietary fat to human cancers of the breast, colon, and prostate.[4] And a pile of recent studies indicate that dietary fat probably plays a role in hundreds of different cancers.[5] Kicking the fat habit is a big step in your cancer prevention program.

Fat and Breast Cancer

Breast cancer is the most feared and the most frequently occurring cancer in American and Canadian women. If you avoid it, pat yourself on the back. Most likely you have protected yourself because, as we covered earlier in the twin studies, diet and lifestyle are by far the biggest factors in this form of cancer.

The wide variation in breast cancer rates worldwide also indicates that diet strongly influences breast cancer. The American diet and other Western diets that cause overweight, especially during postmenopausal years, increase breast cancer risk dramatically. When women with low body mass from countries with low rates of breast cancer, such as Japan, move to the continental US and adopt its much higher fat diet, within two years their breast cancer rates rise to the grim reaper level of Americans.[6]

You can easily dodge the reaper's scythe. Take cystic breast disease for example. Areas of dense breast tissue of many different kinds, lumped together under the label of cysts, are an accepted sign of increased risk of breast cancer. The *Canadian Diet and Breast Cancer Prevention Study* recruited 817 women with dense tissue in more than 50% of the breast area. They were randomly assigned to a group that was taught to reduce dietary fat to less than 21% of calories and a control group whose members were left to fend for themselves. All these women were aware of the cancer risk of fat, so even the control group ate a diet averaging only 32% fat. Mammograms of all subjects were taken at the start and compared with those taken two years later.

Results showed that two years on the low-fat diet significantly reduced the area of dense breast tissue. Even though the control group ate a diet considerably lower in fat (32%) than the American average (34–41%), their dense breast tissue remained as high as ever.[7] Low fat is the way to go.

Because of the evidence linking high levels of the estrogen estradiol to breast cancer, the same researchers also measured sex hormones in these groups of women. After two years, the low-fat group had 20% lower estradiol levels than the control group.[8] These studies are representative of a huge pile of evidence, pointing strongly to a low-fat diet as potent protection against breast cancer, both because of its effects in helping to reduce body fat and its effects in keeping estrogen under control.

Fat and Prostate Cancer

If you feed male mice the typical high-fat American diet, they develop prostate disease. Medical scientists have shown this result repeatedly for the last 40 years. Yet we keep on proving it again and again in the hope that eventually the public will get the message. I have documented it in detail in the book *Protect Your Prostate*.[9] The message is: prostatic hypertrophy and eventually prostate cancer are mostly caused by what you eat.

In one recent study, researchers at Sloan-Kettering Cancer Center in New York fed mice the average American diet for just 16 weeks. In that brief period, the mice developed overgrowth of cells in the prostate. Control mice fed standard laboratory mouse chow showed no prostate abnormalities. The crucial difference between these diets was the higher saturated fat content of the food.[10]

Human studies show the same findings. Dr. A. Whittemore and colleagues at Stanford University School of Medicine in California examined the association of fat intake and prostate cancer in African-Americans (highest risk ethnic group), whites (high risk) and Asian-Americans (low risk) in Los Angeles, San Francisco, and Hawaii in the US, and Vancouver and Toronto in Canada. They compared 1,600 patients with prostate cancer against 1,600 healthy controls for 5 years.

In all patient groups, prostate cancer was strongly linked to saturated fat intake. The African-Americans, who had the highest risk for prostate disease, ate the most saturated fat. The Asian-Americans, who had the lowest risk, ate the least saturated fat.[11]

For all men, removing saturated fats from your diet is crucial for cancer prevention. Prostate cancer is a very slow-growing disease and may be present but not bother you lifelong, unless you speed its progression. Saturated fat can make prostate cancer grow like a weed.

Representative evidence comes from Dr. I. Bairati and team at Laval University in Quebec. They showed that prostate cancer grows more rapidly and aggressively in direct proportion to the amount of saturated fats in the patient's diet.[12] If you want to keep prostate disease at bay, get your fat intake below 25% of total calories, with saturated fats below 10% — and keep it there lifelong.

In this short account, I can't cite even a fraction of the other supporting studies now piled on our desks. But perhaps the summary statement of a leading prostate cancer specialist will help convince you. Dr. William Fair of the Memorial Sloan-Kettering Cancer Center in New York put it this way:

> *We can take a man with a high PSA, put him on a diet containing only 15% fat calories, and watch his PSA drop by 20% in three months.*[13]

Where's the Fat?

Saturated fats are easy to spot in meats and dairy products. But many folk do not realize that vegetable oils can be even worse. Once the vegetable fat is hydrogenated to make margarine, cooking oils, and baked goods, it changes to saturated and trans fats. We detail the problems of processed vegetable oils in our forthcoming book, *Essential Fats*.[14]

With a few simple rules of thumb, you can lower your fat intake dramatically. First, become an avid label reader for all packaged and processed foods. Refuse to buy any packaged food that does not give the fat content. Fat content is given by weight, so add a zero to the fat figure to get the approximate calories of fat. Then find the total calories per serving on the label. If the fat calories are more than a quarter of the total calories, leave it on the supermarket shelf.

Take plain vanilla ice cream for an example. Fat content is 8 grams per serving. Add a zero to get 80 fat calories per serving. Total calories per serving is 160. Fat content, therefore, is 160 divided by 80, a huge 50%. Not an acceptable food for regular use, if you want to prevent cancer.

Contrast this with low-fat frozen yogurt, which today can be made to taste as good as ice cream. Fat content is 2 grams per serving. Add a zero to get 20 fat calories. Total calories per serving is 110. Fat content, therefore, is 110 divided by 20, only 18%. This is a good low-fat food.

The Fat in Meat and Dairy

Most of our meat does not come with the fat content labeled. All fish is fine because fish fats are predominantly unsaturated. Poultry is also fine, as long as you avoid the skin and eat only the white meat. The leg meat of chicken, turkey, and duck is much higher in saturated fat. Lean lamb and veal is fine for occasional use. Eggs are also okay occasionally, and even for regular use if you make your omelets and scrambled eggs from five egg whites and only one egg yolk. You still get all the taste and almost all the protein, but only 20% of the fat.

Cheese is mostly high fat, but for occasional use you can buy low-fat cottage cheese, farmer cheese and hoop cheese, and even some part-skim milk hard cheeses that are lower in fat. Another strategy is to buy high-tasting cheeses such as Stilton, which give you all the taste and satisfaction with a much smaller portion than regular cheddar.

Don't be fooled by slick labeling, such as the big headlines on some packaged meat products that proclaim "90% fat free." Looks like it's only 10% fat. That's just advertising baloney on the bologna. The label figure states fat **by percentage of weight**, which is the legally allowed description on these products. When you work out the percentage of fat calories, the fat just oozes.

Even the traditional low-fat turkey can be rolling in fat. Here are the numbers for a popular brand of "90% fat-free" turkey roll.

Water weight	70%
Fat weight	10%
Protein Weight	20%

The water has zero calories, the fat is 9 calories per gram and the protein is 4 calories per gram. So, in an average 100 gram serving you get:

Total Calories	170
Water: 70 grams	0 calories
Fat: 10 grams	90 calories
Protein: 20 grams	80 calories
Fat calories	90/170 = 53%

This supposed 90% fat-free turkey roll is a whopping 53% fat. That's a higher fat food than regular ice cream.

Keep your calories from fat below 25% of total calories and avoid saturated and trans fats like the plague. It's a great preventive strategy against cancer and has the added benefits of reducing risks of obesity and heart disease.

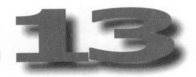

Fiber Prevents Cancer

America and Canada have very high rates of colon and rectal cancers. The American Cancer Society predicts over 148,600 new cases for 2006 and 55,170 deaths.[1] The latest science indicates that ***almost all of these cancers are caused by faulty nutrition***.

The top British medical journal *Lancet* published a huge analysis of diet and colon and rectal cancers in twenty different countries. It shows, unequivocally, that all countries with a high incidence of colorectal cancers eat a high-fat, low-fiber diet. Populations with a low incidence of colorectal cancers all eat a low-fat, high-fiber diet.[2] Uruguay and Argentina, for example, both eat a high beef, low-fiber diet like America. Both have enormous rates of colorectal cancers. Neighboring South American countries that have small meat supplies and eat more vegetables and grains have very low rates.[2]

Is It the Fat or the Fiber?

Colon and rectal cancers develop from many interrelated causes, not just the fat level in the diet. Fiber is a key factor. The body expels many carcinogens in feces. The longer these carcinogens remain in the bowel, the greater the risk they will cause cancerous changes in the bowel lining. A high-fiber diet can reduce the transit time of feces by up to 50%.[3]

Fiber also acts to bind carcinogens in the intestines, making them less active and giving them less access to the intestinal wall. It also assists in maintaining healthy intestinal flora so that they produce fewer carcinogens.[4, 5] Remember, the total weight of flora in your gut, including some 40 different types of beneficial bacteria, is about three pounds, about the same weight as your brain. In healthy folk this essential population lives in balanced harmony and facilitates nutrient absorption, waste elimination, and a host of other body functions. But it can get out of whack, which happens every time you have to take an antibiotic for example. Or one normal form of flora, such as *candida*, can grow out of control, creating mayhem throughout the body. Fiber acts like the police force to control civic unrest in intestinal city.[6]

Another important function of fiber is to control bile acids in the gut. Your liver excretes bile acids into the intestines via the bile duct for elimination. Intestinal bacteria act on these acids, in combination with food wastes, to produce carcinogens. These carcinogens then attack the walls of the bowel. By absorbing bile acids and by speeding transit time, a high-fiber diet reduces this risk substantially.[6]

Reversing Colorectal Cancer

Studies by the National Cancer Institute suggest that fiber is not only preventative, but can even *reverse* developing colorectal cancer. In one recent trial, patients with pre-cancerous polyps in the rectal area were split into two groups. One group ate high-fiber cereal twice daily, containing a daily total of 22.5 grams of fiber, mostly insoluble wheat bran. The other group ate a similar looking cereal that was low in fiber. After four years, results showed clearly that the pre-cancerous polyps of the low-fiber group continued to develop towards cancer. The high-fiber group had fewer and smaller polyps at the end of the study than at the beginning.[7]

Eat Your Veggies

Vegetables are a great fiber source. Many epidemiological studies show that high consumption of vegetables is associated with very low risk of colorectal cancer. Data from the Seven Countries Study, following 12,763 men, aged between 40–59 from 1960 onwards, show that those who eat a low-fiber diet have much higher rates of death from colorectal cancer. An increase of only 10 grams of fiber daily reduced 25-year risk of death from colorectal cancer by 33%.[8] That's big protection.

The National Cancer Institute recommends 25–35 grams of fiber daily.[9] Few Americans or Canadians get that much. The Colgan Institute recommends that you increase your fiber intake as much as possible. Here to help you is Table 13.1 showing servings of foods that contain 10 grams of fiber. Your cancer prevention strategy is to eat three servings from this list every day.

Table 13.1. Colgan Institute Fiber 10

Each item contains about 10 grams of dietary fiber.*

Grains	Vegetables & Seeds	Fruits
½ cup All Bran	½ cup mixed beans	1 cup blueberries
1 cup old-fashioned oatmeal	½ cup peas or lentils	1½ cups blackberries
1 cup mixed whole grains	1 cup peanuts	1½ cups cherries
1½ cups muesli	1 cup pumpkin seeds	3 bananas
3 slices whole rye bread	1 cup sunflower seeds	3 pears
3 slices pumpernickel	2 cups soy beans	4 apples
4 oz. bag popcorn	2 cups steamed vegetables	4 peaches
6 oatmeal cookies	2 cobs sweet corn	6 oranges
	4 cups mixed salad	10 dried figs
	4 medium carrots	20 dried apricots
	2 cups green leaf salad	20 prunes

* Cereal grains are not the best source of fiber.[10] Compared to vegetables and seeds, fruits are considered "second-best" because of their high sugar content. © Colgan Institute 2006

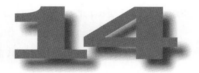

Micronutrients Prevent Cancer

There is a mass of evidence from chemical, cell culture, and animal studies that antioxidant vitamins and related micronutrients are able to prevent cancer and probably slow the progression of existing cancers.[1] Even the highly conservative National Cancer Institute (NCI) can no longer ignore the data. They now state that:

> ... *it is clear that diet can have a significant impact in cancer prevention and control.*[2]

The NCI now supports a wide range of studies that examine common nutrients such as vitamin E and extracts from foods such as polyphenols and isoflavones as cancer preventive agents.[3]

The NCI used to suggest that you can get these vitamins and other nutrients from your diet, especially from fruits and vegetables.

But since 2000, both the American Medical Association and the US National Academy of Sciences have reversed their long-time stance that American food is sufficient and now recommend that Americans take a vitamin and mineral supplement every day. A recent and representative report was published in the *Journal of the American Medical Association* by Robert Fletcher and Kathleen Fairfield of the Harvard Medical School.[4]

Meanwhile, multiple studies show that the general public is woefully deficient in the very foods that NCI say may be essential to protect you from cancer. Since 1971, the US National Health and Nutrition Examination Survey (NHANES) has periodically examined dietary habits in people aged 1–74 in 65 different areas throughout the United States. Back in 1980, the NHANES II survey showed that only 9% of the population ate three or more daily servings of vegetables and two or more servings of fruit.[5] Over 90% of the population got two servings of vegetables or less. These levels are way below the NCI recommendations for a ***minimum*** of five servings per day of fruit and vegetables to prevent cancer.

Surveys in 1987 and 1992 showed little improvement. Although the number of people consuming a high-fat diet decreased, consumption of fruits and vegetables remained pitiful.[6] It seems that most folk still do not understand that failing to eat your veggies is a potent risk for cancer. The evidence is clear. The quarter of the population that eats the least fruits and vegetables has ***double*** the cancer rate, for most types of cancer, of the quarter that eats the most.[6]

Today, after 30 years of effort to educate the public against cancer we have made only a modicum of improvement. Overall, 80% of American children and adolescents and 68% of adults eat less than five portions a day of fruits and vegetables.[7-9] I document these problems in detail in my new book *Nutrition for Champions*.[10] As my friend and colleague Sam Graci always says,

Color your plate.

Don't ever let yourself or your children become a part of the veggie- and fruit-less majority. It's an invitation to cancer.

Essential Nutrient Intakes Dismal

Intake of essential nutrients is equally dismal. Take vitamin A and vitamin C, for example.[10] Only 10% of the population gets the daily recommended levels of vitamin A or C from their diet. The RDA for vitamin C is only 60 mg/day; for vitamin A it is 1000 mcg (3333 i.u.).[11] Even at that low level, 90% of the population is deficient, even at the miniscule levels of intake that make up the US Recommended Dietary Allowances.

Chromium is another essential nutrient required for sugar and fat metabolism and the crucial maintenance of the insulin system. The estimated Safe and Adequate Daily Dietary Intake for chromium is between 50 and 200 mcg per day.[11] Surveys show that the average daily intake in the US and Canada is less than 50 mcg per day.[12] Without sufficient chromium, your body cannot handle sugar. No surprise then that insulin-resistance, adult-onset diabetes, obesity and their related cancers are now epidemic in America.

Zinc is another important nutrient to prevent cancer. As a cell growth regulator it works to prevent cells becoming carcinogenic. The RDA for zinc is 15 mg per day.[11] Data from the NHANES III survey, published in 2000, show nearly two-thirds of the population receive less than the RDA.[8] So, the majority of Americans are not getting enough zinc for average health, certainly not enough to protect them against cancer.

It's the same sad story for numerous other essential nutrients. Researchers examined the diets of participants in the Baltimore Longitudinal Study of Aging to see if they contained adequate amounts of calcium, iron, magnesium, and zinc. Intakes of calcium and magnesium were below the RDA. Thirty percent of participants consumed a deficient amount of iron. Zinc intake was also below the RDA. Remember, these results came from a highly educated, presumably well-nourished group who had been carefully-informed and educated over decades and are willing participants in a world-famous, long-term health study.[13] It doesn't bode well for the rest of us.

Food Degradation

How did our diets go so wrong, from the rough whole grains, organic produce, and lean, free-range meats and wild fish of our forefathers? As we saw in earlier chapters, the research shows clearly that the US food supply has been progressively degraded by heavier and heavier loading of foods with nutritionally empty fats and sugars. Way back in the 1860s, we ate 53% complex carbohydrates, 10% simple sugars and only 25% fats. By 1975 complex carbohydrates had fallen to only 22%, sugars more than doubled to 24%, and fats jumped to 42%.[14] These figures are a gourmet recipe for cancer.

The second major cause of loss of nutrients is soil depletion. With the advent of chemical fertilization, most farm soils in America became over-used and stripped of numerous essential minerals.[15] In farming, the focus is on producing healthy-looking crops, not at all on producing healthy people.

It bears repeating that depleted soils will grow fine-looking crops if fertilized with only nitrogen, phosphorus, and potassium (NPK). But bodies are not vegetables. Human health also requires calcium, chromium, zinc, selenium, iodine, manganese, molybdenum, iron, copper, cobalt, boron, fluoride, nickel, and vanadium. These minerals have been progressively depleted in farm soils since the 1940s.[15]

The third source of loss of nutrients in foods is the hazardous processing journey from field to table.[16] To take a few examples from the American Medical Association's Council on Food and Nutrition, lettuce loses half its vitamin C if kept a mere three days in your refrigerator. Asparagus, broccoli, and green beans lose half their vitamin C in cold storage before they even reach the fridge.[17]

The results are worse if you can foods. Renowned authority on nutrients in food, Dr. Henry Schroeder, has shown repeatedly that canning produces nutritionless pap. Carrots lose 70% of their cobalt; tomatoes lose 80% of their zinc. Canning of green vegetables destroys more than half their contents of B vitamins.[18] Ditch all canned foods if you want to prevent cancer.

You Need Supplementation

We have reviewed five lines of evidence. First, government studies show widespread nutrient deficiencies in American diets. Second, government studies show widespread nutrient deficiencies in American bodies. Third, the composition of the American diet has progressively deteriorated since 1860, so that now it is loaded with nutritionally empty fats and sugars and very low in essential fiber.

Fourth, synthetic fertilization has depleted farm soils of essential minerals. Fifth, modern processing destroys much of the nutrient content of foods. You don't have to be the sharpest knife in the drawer to see that you cannot rely on your food to provide the nutrients to protect you from cancer. Nutrient supplementation is the only sensible way.

The problem is finding appropriate vitamins and minerals. There are hundreds of brands, but only a very few good ones. In America, vitamins come under the food regulations. They are not pharmaceuticals. Anyone can go to a manufacturer, have any formula they like made up, and then sell the hell out of it. No permit is required, no FDA approval, no tests, no qualifications, no certificates, no bona fides at all. For many greedy hands, it's a license to print money.

The Colgan Institute has designed vitamin and mineral formulations as consultants to a huge range of supplement companies, including the two largest in the world. Often the request is to design a pill to a certain price or to fit a certain market niche. We refuse such requests. We design only to fit human health. Even then, by the time the pill hits the market, our original formulation may have been watered down and altered to reduce costs and to increase inclusion of the latest buzz word substance.

Here are one or two of the manufacturer's tricks. Good but expensive forms of minerals, such as ascorbates and picolinates, are replaced by cheap oxides and sulfates that most human bodies can barely absorb or use. Expensive nutrients, such as the B-vitamin biotin, are cut to a few micrograms (millionths of a gram), reducing their action effectively to zero. Other essential nutrients, such as the omega-3 fat alpha-linolenic acid, are left out altogether, because they are difficult to deal with chemically, and reduce the shelf life of the product.

Remember, here we are talking about the good guys, companies prepared to pay high fees to consultants like the Colgan Institute to design the best for them. We never take on the bad guys who litter the market with so-called "miracle" pills, different ones every year. Most of these supplements, especially those sold by multi-level companies and on the Internet, seem to be designed on a napkin in the local greasy spoon, to take advantage of the latest market buzz. Then they are sold with impossible claims at inflated prices for a year or two until the FDA shuts them down.

They rarely catch the con men, however, because the companies usually have offshore owners, beyond the grasp of American authorities. Shut down under one name, they immediately pop up anew under another, complete with shiny new product and even more outlandish claims. Snake-oil carpetbaggers today carry laptops instead and come in Armani suits and rented Mercedes Benz, but their *modus operandi* remains unchanged – fleece the unwary of their money and run.

To help you in your search for quality formulations, you can visit the Colgan Institute website (www.colganinstitute.com) and compare our formulas with formulas that you see in your local health food store or pharmacy. To help you further, Table 13.1 shows a good basic formula based on the goal of preventing cancer.

To prevent cancer you should take a complete nutrient supplement every day. One-a-day pills don't cut it, because you can't fit sufficient nutrient content even into a horse pill. Remember, supplements are the nutrients that used to be abundant in our food, concentrated into pill form. Minerals, especially, take up a lot of room.

Table 13.1. Colgan Institute Basic Daily Vitamin and Mineral Formula

Vitamin A (palmitate)	5,000 IU
Mixed carotenoids (alpha, beta, cryptoxanthin, zeaxanthin)	10,000 IU
Vitamin B1 (thiamin)	100 mg
Vitamin B2 (riboflavin)	50 mg
Vitamin B3 (niacin)	40 mg
(niacinamide)	150 mg
Vitamin B5 (pantothenic acid)	500 mg
Vitamin B6 (pyridoxine)	100 mg
Vitamin B12 (cyanocobalamin)	250 mcg
Vitamin C (ascorbic acid, buffered ascorbates, ascorbyl palmitate)	1,400 mg
Vitamin D3 (cholecalciferous)	400 IU
Vitamin E (d-alpha tocopherol and mixed tocopherols)	400 IU
Betaine (hydrochloride)	150 mg
Bioflavonoids (rose hips, lemon, rutin, hesperidin)	260 mg
Biotin	300 mcg
Boron	1.5 mg
Choline (citrate, bitartrate)	150 mg
Calcium (citrate, ascorbate)	500 mg
Chromium Complex	200 mcg
Copper (chelate)	2 mg
Folic acid	800 mcg
Garlic extract (odorless)	100 mg
Glutamic acid (hydrocholoride)	25 mg
Inositol	100 mg
Iodine (kelp)	200 mcg

L-cysteine & N-acetyl-L-cysteine	150 mg
L-methionine	12.5 mg
Lutein	6 mg
Lycopene	6 mg
Magnesium (aspartate, ascorbate, citrate)	500 mg
Manganese	10 mg
Molybdenum	100 mcg
Para-amino-benzoic-acid	50 mg
Potassium (aspartate)	99 mg
Selenium (selenomethionine)	200 mcg
Vanadium	50 mcg
Zeaxanthin	1 mg
Zinc (chelate)	25 mg
Mixed vegetable, fruit, herb & green food base; includes active flavonoids	800 mg

© Colgan Institute 2003

The biggest pill most people find bearable to swallow weighs 1,300 mg. On its own, 1,000 mg of calcium or 1,000 mg of vitamin C, for example, plus a bit of chalk and protein glue to hold it together, takes the whole pill. So don't believe anyone who tells you that their one (or two)-a-day multis contain all the nutrients you need. They are lying through their teeth.

Never take individual substances either, no matter what the claims. Always buy multiple vitamin/mineral and antioxidant formulas. We see advertisements every day for single nutrients, such as "coral" calcium with lunatic claims that they can cure disease. Codswallop! As we have documented extensively, nutrients work only in synergy with each other, so you need *every* one of them *every* day.[15, 19-21]

And never take your supplements without food. They are food, too, but stripped of the enzyme-activating ingredients in fresh food that are essential to stimulate digestion and assimilation. Without that stimulation, many supplements pass right through the gut, unused. Taken wrongly, even the best nutrient supplements are next to useless to prevent cancer. But taken correctly, complete multiple nutrient supplements can perform miracles.

15

Antioxidants Prevent Cancer

Each breath you take creates damaging residues of oxygen called free radicals. Any form of stress or tension increases free radical production because muscles contract and require more oxygen. Physical work and exercise increase free radicals dramatically because you can use up to 12 times the oxygen used at rest. And numerous stresses in urban and suburban life, such as air pollution, produce their own free radicals. Together these free radical burdens quickly overwhelm your body's inbuilt antioxidant defenses, and cause widespread oxidative damage.[1]

Scientists used to call it the degeneration of aging, as if some mysterious aging clock ticked off our allotted span. Now we know differently. Study after study has shown that any aspect of aging you measure is really measuring damage and disease. Oxidative damage by free radicals is the biggest and most pervasive form of degeneration on Earth. The browning of a cut apple, the rusting of steel, the rotting of meat, and the gradual decay of human flesh all occur primarily by oxidation.[2] Even granite rock slowly oxidizes to dust. To the extent we can prevent this rot, aging and disease cannot occur.

Overwhelming experimental and epidemiological evidence of the last 20 years links oxygen free radicals to many forms of cancer. Oxygen-derived radicals cause damage to membranes, mitochondria and macromolecules including proteins, lipids, and DNA, which distort the design of the body, weaken its defense systems, and allow abnormal cells to proliferate. Any nutrients that disarm these free radicals help us in the fight against cancer.

Potent Antioxidants

Over the last decade, science has made two major advances in knowledge of nutrient antioxidants. First, we now know there are dozens of them, and likely hundreds more waiting to be discovered. Second, although each of the known antioxidants has specific tasks to perform in an ideally functioning body, they all work in precise synergy with each other. If you miss one out, or take too little or too great a quantity of another, it can disrupt the balance and the action of all the rest.

So whenever you see media accounts that this or that antioxidant reduces this or that disease, or is "the master antioxidant," or the "only one you need," remember that the "news" is often a similar level of misinformation as the advertisements which surround it. And whenever you hear a physician admit he now takes vitamin E or vitamin C or some clever sounding chemical, such as idebenone, you know to drive quickly *past* his office if ever you need medical treatment.   If you supplement with one thing, you have to supplement with everything else to maintain the synergy. The first principle is complete nutrition.

We would all be dead of free radical damage tomorrow were it not for the body's production of endogenous antioxidants. Your body makes these itself. The main ones are **superoxide dismutase (SOD)**, **catalase**, and **glutathione**. These antioxidants "quench" free radicals by receiving or donating an electron. This action converts the antioxidant itself into a free radical, although of a less damaging chemical form. Other antioxidants immediately step in to quench the new free radical and also become free radicals, but less damaging again. This chemical oxidation and reduction process continues using a variety of antioxidants, until it ends up as harmless waste products, primarily carbon dioxide and water, which are then excreted from the body via urine, sweat, and breath. Now you know why only a complete supplement of a variety of antioxidants can neutralize oxidative damage.

Antioxidants and Cancer

Many studies demonstrate that antioxidants are much better at *preventing* cancer than curing or treating it.   Modern chemotherapy, radiation, and surgery are frequently unable to treat or cure cancer either, so it is unrealistic to expect simple nutrients to accomplish this very difficult task. The key to cancer will always be prevention.

For cancer prevention, antioxidants work in a wide variety of ways. They can be anti-mutagenic, tumor growth inhibitors, mitochondrial protectors, gene regulators, or hormone regulators.

Different antioxidants also work differently and in different parts of your body. Science is still pretty dumb when trying to measure actions of diverse groups of biochemicals *in vivo*. To find out the exact action of each antioxidant, we still have to examine them one or two at a time. As we discuss examples of these isolation studies, keep in mind that they, and you, rely for success on the whole antioxidant team.

Vitamin A

Long known for its beneficial effects on skin and mucous membranes, vitamin A is especially effective at protecting the membranes of the colon. In representative animal studies, rats supplemented with vitamin A show significantly reduced polyps of the colon compared with controls.[3] This preventive effect of vitamin A is probably due to direct protection of colon epithelial cells (the living cells just below the surface). Remember, 80% of cancers occur outside the body, either on the skin or in the open tube that runs from mouth to anus.

Vitamin A also works inside the body. Recent studies looked at the effect of the retinyl acetate form of vitamin A, plus melatonin, on rat mammary cancer induced with the carcinogen N-methyl-N-nitrosourea. This study is a good example of the interaction of antioxidants. Results showed that there were significantly fewer tumors in the group treated with **both** retinyl acetate and melatonin, compared with retinyl acetate alone.[4]

It often depends on the particular carcinogen, however. In further studies, researchers induced mammary tumors using the carcinogen 9,10-dimethyl-1,2-benzanthracene (DMBA). Retinyl acetate proved more effective ***alone*** than when combined with melatonin.[5] In all of these studies, of course, many other antioxidants were involved both from the diet and made in the body. Our analytic tools restrict the focus of measurement to one or two. At the Colgan Institute, we use 5,000–10,000 IU of vitamin A every day.

Vitamin C

Dr. Linus Pauling caused apoplexy in academic halls when he first proposed using large supplements of vitamin C in the 1960s.[6] Since then, many experts like Dr. Bruce Ames have confirmed Pauling's work.[7] More than 100 controlled studies now show strong effects of vitamin C in prevention of a variety of cancers, including hormone-based cancers of the breast, endometrium, and prostate.[8] Studies of the killing action of vitamin C on prostate cancer cell lines, have emphasized the antioxidant action of the nutrient and have even shown how to enhance this action up to 20 times by the addition of vitamin K.[9]

Provided you take enough, the body maintains high levels of the ascorbic acid form of vitamin C in the gastric mucosa. Researchers now believe that this vitamin concentration plays an important role in the prevention of colon cancer.[10] We know, for example, that some gut cancers are caused by processed foods that contain nitrates and nitrites. These preservatives become potent carcinogens by forming substances called **nitrosamines**. One way that vitamin C prevents colon cancers is by stopping nitrosamines from forming.[11]

Vitamin C also protects your genetic code. A representative study looked at the role of vitamin C and glutamine in protecting chromosomes from changes caused by the carcinogenic agent doxorubicin (DXR). Results showed that both these nutrients significantly reduced damage to chromosomes.[12]

Vitamin C also protects the cervix. In a series of representative studies, researchers induced cervical cancer in mice, using the carcinogen methylcholoanthrene (MCA). Ascorbic acid was given daily in drinking water for different periods. Results showed that, of a group given the ascorbic acid during the initial phase and throughout the introduction of the carcinogen, 33% developed tumors. Twice as many (66%) developed tumors when given the ascorbic acid only *after* the introduction of the MCA. For best effect, you have to have the vitamin C in your body before the carcinogen attacks.[14]

Other studies indicate that the anti-cancer effect of vitamin C involves multiple mechanisms in addition to its antioxidant action. These include enhancing immune system action against cancer, neutralizing carcinogenic substances, and destroying viruses and other infectious agents that promote cancer or speed its growth. Vitamin C also stimulates collagen formation to surround and encapsulate tumors to inhibit their progression.[8] It's a critical player on your antioxidant defense team. We use 2–4 grams of mixed ascorbates every day.

Vitamin E

Strong evidence supports vitamin E in cancer prevention. In a massive study, Dr. P. Knekt and colleagues in Finland followed 21,000 men for 10 years. Men with high vitamin E intake and high blood levels of vitamin E had a 30% lower risk *for all types of cancer*.[13]

In a second study, Dr. Knekt followed 15,000 women for eight years. All were initially free of cancer. During the follow-up, women with high serum vitamin E developed 60% fewer cancers than women with low serum vitamin E.[14] Folk would be scrambling to buy any car safety device that would reduce risk of injury in accidents by 60%, no matter what the price. Yet most folk still ignore inexpensive, non-toxic vitamin E that can provide the same potent protection against cancer. Don't be one of them.

Recent research from Russia indicates that, because of its strong antioxidant action in lipids, vitamin E supplementation is also effective in prevention of prostate disease. In a controlled trial using long-term supplementation with alpha-tocopherol, results showed a dramatic reduction in prostate cancer incidence and mortality in men using vitamin E.[15]

Vitamin E even protects the skin. Recent studies show that vitamin E compounds put into sunscreens help prevent DNA photo-damage from ultra-violet light.[16] Putting antioxidants on your skin does not prevent wrinkles despite the claims of cosmetic conglomerates. But it can prevent skin damage a lot more serious than that "map of days outworn." We use vitamin E, plus mixed tocopherols and tocotrienols, in amounts of 800–1,600 IU per day.

Glutathione

L-glutathione is one of your main endogenous antioxidants. The body makes glutathione from the amino acids l-cysteine, glutamic acid, and l-glycine. Glutathione is probably our main cellular defense against alkylating and oxidative carcinogens. Unfortunately, glutathione levels decline with aging. But older people who manage to maintain high blood levels of glutathione suffer fewer cancers than those with the usual low levels. [17]

New evidence shows that depletion of glutathione permits progression of certain cancers.[17,18] As many cancers are slow-growing, over decades before they become detectable as tumors, you should do everything to keep glutathione high to stem cancer progression. Oral glutathione itself is poorly absorbed by humans, but supplements of n-acetyl cysteine, a precursor of glutathione, raise blood levels of glutathione very nicely. We use 200–400 mg every day.

Selenium

The element selenium was recognized only 40 years ago as being essential in the nutrition of animals and humans. It is a component of a number of enzymes in which it occurs as the amino acid selenocysteine. Selenium has other roles, also. Many studies show that it inhibits the development of tumors in a variety of animal models of cancer. Following this lead, recent studies show that supplemental selenium in human diets may reduce cancer risk.[19]

Selenium operates by various mechanisms to prevent cancer, depending on dosage, the chemical form of the selenium, and the nature of the carcinogen. It is a growth modulator that helps to prevent the transformation of cells.[20] In addition, it inhibits the replication of tumor viruses, it protects DNA against carcinogen-induced damage, and it stops the proliferation of blood vessels in tumor cells.[21] Selenium supplementation has been found beneficial in breast,[21] lung,[22] and prostate[23] cancer. It is a powerful antioxidant in your armor against cancer.

Unfortunately, selenium is now deficient in most soils worldwide.[24] Way back in 1980, I documented its deficiency in the soils of 10 states producing food in the US.[24] As a result most food chains contain inadequate selenium.[25]

Some vegetables are better at gathering selenium, even when it is scarce. Members of the *Allium* genus (onions and garlic) are seleniferous. That is, they readily uptake inorganic selenium from the soil and incorporate it into bioactive chemicals. The brassicas (cabbage, broccoli, and cauliflower) are also good at selenium uptake. Make these a regular part of your diet.

We also supplement with the organic form of selenium, **selenomethionine,** in amounts of 200–800 mcg per day. Note that the dose is in micrograms (millionths of a gram) *not* milligrams (thousandths of a gram). So we are talking 0.2–0.8 milligrams.

Coenzyme Q10

Your body can't make coenzyme Q10 completely. It has to derive it from coenzyme Q, which occurs widely in foods, from where it gets its common name ubiquinone. Despite this abundance, the level of coenzyme Q10 declines in your body with age. This decline has now been traced to decline of an enzyme in the liver that converts CoQ to CoQ10.[26]

When tested in animals, Coenzyme Q10 has both anti-cancer and immune system enhancing properties.[27] It is an essential cofactor of the electron transport chain, as well as a potent free radical scavenger in lipids and mitochondrial membranes. Recent research shows it to have strong protective effects against degenerative diseases of the brain.[27, 28] The best form of Co Q10 is **idebenone**, used widely in Europe but still uncommon in the US. You can obtain idebenone from www.antiaging-systems.com. We use doses of 20–40 mg per day.

Melatonin

Most folk are familiar with melatonin in its role as a "sleeping pill." Pineal gland output of melatonin is part of your circadian rhythm of hormone production in concert with the sleep/wake cycle. It maintains the synchrony of both sleep and the hormone cascade. Melatonin declines rapidly with usual aging.[29]

Besides restoring the circadian synchrony of your hormones, many new studies show further benefits of supplemental melatonin. First, it is a powerful brain antioxidant that inhibits brain aging by destroying free radicals.[29] Second, studies on melatonin as an anticarcinogen show that it aids other antioxidants in their roles, as well as playing multiple roles of its own.

A representative study examined the role of melatonin in colon carcinogenesis.[30] Researchers induced colon cancer in rats. Results demonstrated that supplemental melatonin strongly inhibited cancer development. It is likely that melatonin works in this cancer by two mechanisms. First, it strengthens the immune system. Second, it has direct radical scavenging effects that inhibit tumor growth.[31]

You don't need much melatonin. The form we recommend is a sublingual pill taken just before bed. Dosage of 1-3 mg is sufficient. Not a lot, but without it your sleep and your hormones are disturbed, and cancer is always lurking, ready to attack at any sign of bodily weakness.

Mitochondrial Antioxidants

Now we come to the most important part of antioxidant protection against cancer, a part that you will not likely have heard of yet, as the science still has to break through the media ignorance barrier. About 90% of free radicals made in your body are generated by the energy process at the **mitochondria**. These microscopic structures in your cells produce your basic energy molecule, **adenosine triphosphate,** from food which combines with the oxygen you breathe to release energy. The process is far from perfect. Most of the damage to your mitochondria and the cells enclosing them occurs from free radicals produced by the chemical reactions themselves or by molecules of oxygen that escape mitochondrial regulation.

Between ages 25 and 60, the mitochondria become so damaged in the average person that energy production declines *by half.* These weakened cells are easy prey for cancer and other degenerative diseases. Numerous scientists have developed Denman Harmon's early discoveries about free radicals in the 1950s to show clearly that mitochondrial oxidative damage is the main process by which we age and die.[32]

Cancer is the second largest killer in Westernized nations, beaten only narrowly by cardiovascular disease. We know now that the mitochondrial damage that weakens cells and enables cancers to invade the body is the major process underlying this terrible group of diseases. Protecting your mitochondria from oxidative damage is a prime goal in prevention of cancer.

The big problem is none of the common nutrient antioxidants have any effect on mitochondrial free radicals because they cannot get inside your cells. As Harmon first proposed in 1972, you have to use substances that normally occur inside cells. Mitochondria can be protected only by mitochondrial antioxidants.[33]

What are these substances? I introduced five mitochondrial antioxidants in Chapter 4: R+ lipoic acid, acetyl-l-carnitine, L-carnosine, idebenone, and n-acetyl cysteine.   Idebenone is a derivative of coenzyme Q10, which we have already discussed. It works as both an extra-cellular and intracellular antioxidant. Glutathione, too, works both outside and inside our cells and can be included in our list of mitochondrial antioxidants.

Because mitochondrial antioxidants have only a recent commercial history and are unknown to most of the public, we should document the actions and effects of these substances to yield a credible account.   But there is no space in this small book to do so.   The best we can do is refer the reader to our new book, *Brain Power*,[34] which provides the necessary documentation.   Here we will simply state the case for three of these nutrients, with citations, and hope it is enough.

R+ Lipoic Acid

The first mitochondrial protector is **R+ lipoic acid**.   This is not the alpha lipoic acid currently sold in pharmacies and health food stores, which is the R+S- lipoic acid and is virtually useless.   R+ lipoic acid is the naturally occurring form which has the correct chemical keys to fit your mitochondrial locks.

There are now many studies showing how R+ lipoic acid protects mitochondria.   But because the data are complex and very recent, few simplified accounts have yet been written, so this huge advance in science has yet to stir the media.   Representative studies show reversal of mitochondrial decay, improved mitochondrial function, reduction in oxidative damage to cell proteins and lipids, and inhibition of cell aging.[35, 36] We use 300–600 mg of R+ lipoic acid every day.

Acetyl-l-carnitine

When R+ lipoic acid is combined with a second naturally occurring mitochondrial metabolite called **acetyl-l-carnitine,** results really shine.[36] This is not the l-carnitine commonly sold in stores. Only the acetylated form can pass into cells easily and protect intracellular function. We use 500–2,000 mg of acetyl-l-carnitine every day.

CDP-Choline

The third mitochondrial antioxidant is **cytidine 5-diphosphate-choline (CDP-choline)**. It inhibits oxidative damage in lipids and protects an essential component of the mitochondrial membrane called **cardiolipin**. It also stimulates production of the endogenous antioxidant glutathione.[37] We use 500–1,000 mg of CDP-choline every day.

Summary

Many people still think it "unnatural" to take pills all your life. It is equally unnatural to buy your food in packets from the supermarket rather than grow it. It is also unnatural to live in synthetic, man-made, toxic environments, where unnatural carcinogenic fumes, pesticides and other unnatural additives assault us every day in our food, water, and air. Providing your body with a continuous supply of the nutrients necessary to combat these unnatural toxins is a handsome return for swallowing a few pills.

I have reviewed some representative findings of antioxidant effects against cancer. The strongest evidence is for vitamins, A, C, and E; n-acetyl cysteine as a precursor of the endogenous antioxidant glutathione; coenzyme Q10; melatonin; R+ lipoic acid; acetyl-l-carnitine; and CDP-choline. Amounts we use at the Colgan Institute are given in Table 15.1. All should form part of a complete daily supplement. Additional antioxidant effects of flavonoids and carotenoids are covered ahead. Our cancer prevention armor is starting to take shape.

Table 15.1. Antioxidant Supplements To Prevent Cancer

Nutrient	Daily Range
Vitamin A	5000 – 10,000 IU
Vitamin C	2 – 4 grams
Vitamin E	800 – 1600 IU
N-acetyl cysteine	200 – 400 mg
Selenomethionine	0.2 – 0.8 mg
Melatonin	1 – 3 mg
R+ lipoic acid	300 – 600 mg
Acetyl-l-carnitine	500 – 2000 mg
CDP-choline	500 – 1000 mg

© Colgan Institute 2006

16

Flavonoids Prevent Cancer

As documented in earlier chapters, vegetables are one of the most important weapons against cancer. Most people react to such a statement with, "Sure, vegetables are good for you." But until the scientific discoveries of the last decade, we did not realize just how good. Now we know that simple everyday items, like cabbage, broccoli, and carrots, contain natural substances that are more powerful inhibitors of cancer than all the high-tech chemotherapy, radiation therapy, and cancer surgery put together.

Better yet, they were all in the environment four million years ago when the human body was evolving. So, unlike the chemotherapy and radiation therapy developed over the last 100 years, which are highly toxic, the human system had the millions of years necessary to evolve mechanisms to utilize these natural chemicals as non-toxic nutrients. As we will see, constituents of vegetables are likely to prove the biggest advance against cancer of the 21ˢᵗ century. Let's look at some representative evidence.

Recent studies have identified numerous flavonoids in produce that inhibit cancer cell proliferation. The major classes of flavonoids are phenols, indoles, isoflavones, coumarins, and aromatic isothiocyanates.[1] We will examine a few examples of each.

Phenols

Numerous phenols occur in edible plants. A well-known example is 4-hydroxy-3-methoxy cinnamic acid. It is widely sold as a sports supplement under the popular name of **ferulic acid**. It is the major active substance in **gamma oryzanol**, a compound extracted from rice bran oil.

Ferulic acid and at least two other plant phenols inhibit stomach cancer induced in mice.[2] In representative *in vivo* and *in vitro* experiments, researchers tested the phenols **ellagic acid**, **tannic acid**, **caffeic acid**, and ferulic acid to see if they would inhibit tumors in their initial phase of growth. Ferulic acid, tannic acid, and caffeic acid were all found to be strong tumor growth inhibitors.[3]

Another class of phenols is found in green and black tea. Tea is processed differently in different parts of the world to give green tea (20%), black tea (78%) or oolong tea (2%). Numerous cell and animal studies demonstrate the potency of tea against various mutagens (substances that cause cells to mutate into precursors of cancer cells).[4] Studies also show anti-carcinogenic activity of tea phenols in transplantable tumors, carcinogen-induced tumors in digestive organs, mammary glands, liver cancers, lung cancers, skin tumors, leukemia, and tumor promotion and metastasis.[4] Tea is not just a drink for old ladies in the afternoon. It is an essential part of your armor against cancer.

Green tea is especially effective. One recent study on 472 patients found that consumption of green tea was linked to reduced lymph node metastases among pre-menopausal women with Stage I and Stage II breast cancer.[5] The researchers also reported that increased consumption of green tea was correlated with reduced recurrence of breast cancer.

Tea consumption also helps inhibit tumors of the digestive tract. In a study using rats with artificially-induced esophagus tumors, both green and black tea reduced the incidence of tumors.[6] The group that was given green and black tea during the initial treatment with the carcinogen had a 70% reduction in tumor growth over controls. The group given the tea after tumor growth had occurred had a 55% reduction in tumors over controls. Get the green tea habit *before* the cancer occurs. Prevention is always the way.

Green tea is also good news for men. The enzyme ornithine decarboxylase is high in men with prostate cancer.[7] This enzyme is expressed by an androgen-responsive gene, and the androgenic stimulation regulates the development and growth of both normal and tumorigenic prostate cells. Research using both *in vitro* (test-tube) and *in vivo* models (mice) shows that green tea inhibits tumor formation by controlling the amount of ornithine decarboxylase uptake by cells.[8]

Green tea may help even with skin cancer. An *in vivo* study using mice evaluated the protective effect of drinking green tea against the change of normal cells to papillomas, and consequently to squamous cell carcinomas. The researchers concluded that green tea phenols reduce skin cancer risk.[9]

Another major class of phenols is the **proanthocyanidins** found in pine bark, grape seeds, and bilberry leaves. These have received a lot of press and are important antioxidants and anti-inflammatories. Recent research shows them to be promising anti-tumor substances, too.[10] Other promising polyphenols are **resveratrol** and **quercetin** found in vegetables, citrus fruits, and red grapes.[11]

Indoles

Indoles occur naturally in cruciferous vegetables such as cabbage, cauliflower, broccoli, and brussel sprouts. The best known of the indoles is **indole-3-carbinol**.

In a representative study, 60 women at increased risk for breast cancer were enrolled in a placebo-controlled, double-blind dose-ranging chemoprevention study. Results showed that indole-3-carbinol, at a minimum effective dose of 300 mg per day, is a promising preventive agent against breast cancer.[12]

The chemotherapy drug **tamoxifen** is the treatment of choice for many breast cancers. But it is effective in less than 50% of cases. A recent study found that a combination of indole-3-carbinol and tamoxifen works to inhibit the growth of estrogen-dependent breast cancer more effectively than either substance alone.[13]

When to take the indole-3-carbinol is a crucial variable in preventing cancer. A recent study on rats examined indole-3-carbinol's ability to inhibit development of liver cancer, when given either before or after exposure to a carcinogen.[14] Animals that were pretreated with indole-3-carbinol for two weeks prior to administration of the carcinogen, and continued to receive it during exposure to the carcinogen, were protected from development of cancerous lesions.

Animals who did not receive it prior to exposure to the carcinogen did not experience any protective effect. This study illustrates how important it is to maintain these substances in your body all the time for effective protection against cancer.

Isoflavones

The most researched isoflavones are **genistein** and **diadzein** extracted from soy. Because the chemical structure of these compounds is similar to estradiol, they are also called **phytoestrogens**. These soy isoflavones likely exert cancer preventive effects by reducing estrogen synthesis and by altering metabolism to avoid producing the more toxic metabolites of estrogen.[15]

A large population-based case-control study has demonstrated that women with a high intake of soy foods reduce their risk of breast cancer.[16] Another experiment on human mammary cells found that indole-3-carbinol, tea polyphenols, and the soy isoflavone genistein all inhibited cancer cell proliferation.[17]

Genistein also plays a role in reducing risk of prostate cancer. Significant levels of genistein occur in human prostatic fluid. Representative studies showed that genistein affects gene regulation, which results in the inhibition of cell growth and ultimate demise of tumor cells.[18]

Soy isoflavones also inhibit bladder cancer. One representative study using mice with induced bladder cancer found that those treated with soy isoflavones showed a reduction in tumor volume of 48% compared with controls.[19] Researchers found that the soy reduced angiogenesis, (growth of blood supply to the tumor), increased tumor cell death, and reduced tumor proliferation, while having no adverse effect on normal bladder cells.

New research is also examining the role of genistein in lung cancer. Lung cancer is the leading cause of cancer-related death in the world, with increasing incidence in many developed countries. A recent study investigated cell growth inhibition and cell death by genistein in non-small lung cancer cells. Researchers concluded that genistein may act as an anti-cancer agent because of its modulation of cell growth and cell death.[20] Soy isoflavones provide tough, non-toxic, yet inexpensive, armor against cancer.

Coumarins

The most studied herbal containing coumarins is the spice turmeric. The chemical structure of curcumin was determined in 1910, but it was not until the 1970s that researchers began to document the potential benefits of curcuminoid compounds. A recent study, representative of the last 20 years of evidence, evaluated the chemopreventive effects of the most active coumarin, curcumin, on radiation-induced tumors in rat mammary glands. Sixty-four pregnant rats received whole body irradiation at day 20 of pregnancy. After weaning they were divided into two groups. The control group was fed a basic diet and then implanted with a DES pellet for 1 year. Eighty-four percent developed mammary tumors. A second group was fed a diet containing 1% curcumin, beginning immediately after weaning and also received a DES pellet. Tumor incidence was reduced to 28% in this group.[21] That's a huge protective effect.

Further studies show that curcumin inhibits chemically-induced carcinogenesis of the skin, stomach, and colon. One typical study investigated whether curcumin is chemopreventive when administered later in the pre-malignant stage during promotion and progression of colon cancer. The researchers found that, even when the cancer process was well under way, curcumin suppressed the incidence and multiplicity of both invasive and non-invasive carcinomas of the colon.[22]

Isothiocyanates

Isothiocyanates occur in many edible plants, most commonly in cruciferous vegetables.   Isothiocyanates block cancer progress in animal models by inhibiting carcinogen activation and by accelerating the inactivation of carcinogens.[23, 24]

A recent study using an animal model suggests that **phenethyl isothiocyanate** may be a strong chemopreventive agent for lung cancer.[25] This isothiocyanate blocks the metabolic activation of one particular carcinogen and aids in its excretion via the urinary tract.

Isothiocyantes also inhibit the development of esophageal tumors. In studies using animal models, dietary concentrations of isothiocyantes reduced the incidence and multiplicity of induced esophageal tumors by more than 95%.[26]   Can't get much better than that.

There are many more flavonoid susbstances in fruits and vegetables. We have looked at only a few of them. Some are only now being researched, while others, like the citrus flavonoids in citrus fruits, we have known about for decades.   In order to protect yourself against cancer, eat a wide variety of fresh fruits and vegetables every day and, whenever possible, make sure they are organic. Also, ensure that your daily supplements contain at least three grams of a wide variety of mixed flavonoids. The flavonoids which have the strongest evidence supporting their use against cancer are given in Table 16.1 below. No one knows the ideal amounts to take. We have derived the figures given from a summary of doses found effective in the experimental studies referenced, plus our database of similar controlled research.

Table 16.1. Flavonoids To Prevent Cancer

Flavonoids	Daily Amount
Ferulic acid	200 mg
Tea phenols	500 mg
Pine, grape and bilberry proanthocyanidins	500 mg
Indole-3-carbinol	300 mg
Soy isoflavones genistein & diadzein	50 mg
Curcumin (with piperine)	300 mg
Crucifer isothiocyanates	400 mg

© Colgan Institute 2006

Carotenoids Prevent Cancer

Ever wondered where the glorious colors of fall come from? The hundreds of different reds, yellows, and oranges that provide our annual treat are all carotenoids. They form in leaves to protect them from ultra-violet radiation while they do their job of gathering light to grow the tree. They are finally revealed in deciduous trees in fall, as their green chlorophyll "blood" ceases to flow.

Science has identified over 600 of these pigmented compounds, but until recently, they were thought of little importance. Beta-carotene did become a popular supplement in the 1980s, but most of it used in research at that time was synthetic beta-carotene, which has different chemical properties than the natural compound. So results were generally negative, and it fell into disfavor. Recent science has proven that synthetic beta-carotene simply doesn't work.[1]

Today we know that the six carotenoids which occur in the greatest concentration in the human body are major players in the game of health. These are alpha-carotene, beta-carotene, lycopene, lutein, zeaxanthin, and cryptoxanthin. Along with vitamin E and other tocopherols and tocotrienols, these carotenoids are now ranked as our main fat-soluble antioxidants.[2]

Some carotenoids, such as beta-carotene, are precursors of vitamin A, but also have strong antioxidant activity of their own. Others, like lycopene, have no vitamin A potential, but exhibit strong activity against singlet oxygen free radicals. Lutein and zeaxanthin are the carotenoids that protect the macular region of the retina, your point of clearest vision. They act to help process light, much as they do in plant leaves, and are also strong antioxidants, essential to maintain your eyes[3] Remember, macular degeneration is the largest single cause of blindness in the US and Canada, strong evidence that our usual diet does not contain sufficient lutein and zeaxanthin.

A mass of human and animal research shows that carotenoids also enhance the immune response. And they protect the skin from damage following exposure to UV radiation. Beta-carotene, in particular, protects against UV-induced suppression of immune responses. We cover carotenoid effects on immunity in Chapter 19 ahead.

High Carotenoids, Low Cancer Risk

Here we are concerned more with the effects of carotenoids against cancer, independent of the immune system. Recent research has uncovered a most important anti-cancer function. To put it in a nutshell, carotenoids enhance communication between cells by increasing the flow of regulatory signals. When normal cells use this enhanced communication to "talk" to cells that have been damaged by carcinogens, it prevents the damaged cells turning malignant. This regulatory communication also inhibits proliferation of cells that have already become malignant.[2] Every day your body produces malignant cells that can proliferate into cancer. Carotenoids provide a strong protective mechanism to keep these cells under control.

Research on cancer confirms the power of carotenoids. More than 60 recent studies show that cancer patients have very low levels of carotenoids. Conversely, people with the highest intakes of carotenoid-rich fruits and vegetables and high blood levels of carotenoids have the lowest risk for numerous types of cancer.

To take a few representative examples, breast cancer risk is dramatically reduced by high levels of beta-carotene and/or lutein and zeaxanthin, even in women with a family history of breast cancer.[4, 5] Cervical cancer risk is much reduced in women with high serum levels of total carotenoids.[6] Beta-carotene levels are low in patients with stomach and digestive tract cancers.[7, 8] In men, those with beta-carotene intake in the highest range have one-third the risk for stomach and digestive tract cancers.[9] High dietary carotenoids and high blood levels of alpha- and beta-carotene, lutein and zeaxanthin also greatly reduce the risk of lung cancer.[10] And a high intake of lycopene reduces risk of prostate cancer.[11]

If that's not enough to convince you, search for information on "carotenoids and cancer" in the *Entrez PubMed* database of the US National Library of Medicine (www.ncbi.nih.gov/entrez/query. fcgi?db=PubMed). Just to read the recent evidence that carotenoids prevent cancer will take you longer than to read this entire book. Most of this work has not hit the public news yet.

Carotenoids from Your Diet

Research shows consistently that it takes higher intakes of carotenoids than are consumed in even a good diet to inhibit cancer. Non-invasive scans, now available widely in clinics across the US and Canada, show average blood levels of total carotenoids of about 20,000 units in people who *report* diets high in carotenoids. This range is now considered too low for protection. A score of 50,000 units plus is probably sufficient. I had the scan done as this book was going to press. The result: 77,000 units of total carotenoids in my blood.

To obtain sufficient carotenoids, select your fruits and vegetables well. A diet that includes daily broccoli, carrots, tomato juice, watermelon, and pink grapefruit provides about 11,000 IU per day of beta-carotene and over 20,000 mcg of other carotenoids. But a diet that includes cabbage, iceberg lettuce, white potato, an apple, and a pear provides less than 1,000 IU of beta-carotene, less than 50 mcg of alpha-carotene, only 350 mcg of lutein and zeaxanthin, and no lycopene or cryptoxanthin. That is way too few carotenoids to protect you.

Tables 17.1 and 17.2 give the carotenoid content of common foods. You can see that orange juice is pathetic, but raw, fresh oranges are great. Red peppers beat the hell out of yellow peppers. Plums, pears, and raspberries have negligible carotenoids, whereas tomatoes are loaded. Cabbage is a poor source, but carrots are overflowing. Iceberg lettuce is useless, but romaine is protective for vision. And with regular spinach, Popeye is unlikely to go blind.

Table 17.1. Carotenoids in Fruit (mcg/100 grams)

All values are for fresh raw fruit unless otherwise indicated.

Fruit	Beta-Carotene	Alpha-Carotene	Lutein Zeaxanthin	Lycopene	Crypto-xanthin	Total Carotenoids
Apple		30				30
Apricot	6,600			65		6,665
Banana	21	5	0	0	0	26
Blueberry	35	0				35
Cantaloupe	1,600	27	40	0	0	1,667
Grapefruit, white	14	8				22
Grapefruit, pink	600	5	12	1,500	12	2,129
Grape, red	39					39
Mango	450	17			11	478
Nectarine	101	0			60	161
Orange juice	4	2	36		15	535
Orange	50	15	190	0	120	375
Papaya	275	0	75	0	760	1110
Peaches	97	1	57	0	24	179
Pear	27	6				33
Pineapple	30					30
Plum	98				16	114
Raspberry	8	12			0	20
Strawberry			5			5
Tangerine	71	14	243	0	485	813
Tomato juice	428	0	60	9,200	0	9,688
Tomato, cooked	300	0	150	4,400	0	4,850
Tomato	393	112	130	3,025	0	3,660
Watermelon	295	0	17	4,900	103	5,315

©Colgan Institute 2006   Blank cells, no value reported.

Table 17.2. Carotenoids in Vegetables (mcg/100 grams)

All values are for fresh raw vegetables unless otherwise indicated.

Vegetable	Beta-Carotene	Alpha-Carotene	Lutein Zeaxanthin	Lycopene	Crypto-xanthin	Total Carotenoids
Asparagus, steamed	495	10				505
Avocado	50	30			35	115
Broccoli, steamed	1,040	0	2,225	0	0	3,265
Cabbage	90					90
Carrot	8,850	4,650				13,500
Celery	150	0	230	0	0	380
Cucumber	31	8				39
Green beans, steamed	550	90	700	0	0	1,340
Kale, steamed	6,200	0	15,800	0	0	22,000
Lettuce, romaine	1,275	0	2,650	0	0	3,925
Lettuce, iceberg	190	2	350	0	0	542
Peas	320	0	1,350	0	0	1,670
Pepper, yellow	120					120
Pepper, green	198	22				220
Pepper, red	2,400	60			2,200	2,660
Potato, sweet, baked	9,500	0	0	0	0	9,500
Potato, white, baked	6					6
Pumpkin, baked	7,000	4,800	0	0	0	7,400
Spinach, cooked	5,250	0	7,000	0	0	12,250
Spinach	600	0	12,000	0	0	12,600
Squash, acorn	490	0	66	0	0	556
Squash, butternut	4,570	1,130				5,700
Squash, zucchini	410	0	2,125	0	0	2,535

©Colgan Institute 2006   Blank cells, no values reported.

To prevent cancer, use these tables to make good food choices. Then add 20,000–30,000 mcg of mixed carotenoid supplements every day. Aim for a constant blood level of at least 50,000 units.

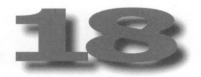

Essential Fats Prevent Cancer

The human body is brilliant at making fat. As dieters know only too bitterly, it can make a barrel of body fat out of any food you eat – carbohydrates, proteins, or fats. It can even turn hormones like insulin into fat.[1] It's a fat-manufacturing plant *par excellence*.

But there are two fats your body cannot make, **linoleic acid** (omega-6) and **alpha-linolenic acid** (omega-3).[2] You must obtain these essential fats from your food. Almost all omega-6 fats come from vegetable oils. So do omega-3 fats, except those in fish oils. Meats and dairy foods contain only miniscule amounts of essential fats.

Essential fats have to be alive to be useful. In other words, they must keep their biological activity potential intact. Most processed fats are dead fats.

Omega-6 and omega-3 fats are essential for oxygen uptake, regulation of blood pressure, formation of hemoglobin, and insulin metabolism. Paradoxically, they are also essential for maintaining a low level of body fat. Even more important, they are the raw materials you need to make all your special fats in the structure of your brain, eyes, ears, testes, ovaries, adrenals, and in the membranes that surround and protect every cell in your body.

Without these two essential fats in your diet, you would become a decaying blob of flesh, progressively losing the ability to think, see, hear, reproduce, or even move a muscle.[2, 3] Whenever your dietary supply of essential fats becomes inadequate, your body degenerates towards that blob.

Even the conservative RDA Handbook recommends a daily intake of about six grams of linoleic acid and two grams of alpha-linolenic acid. That makes your requirement for essential fats larger than for any of the vitamins or minerals.[3] Since these RDA's came out in 1989, new evidence recommends an even larger daily requirement. Very few of us get enough.

Only certified organic, unprocessed oils can provide the two essential fats in the undamaged form that you need. And only a few of these oils provide the fats in anything like the right proportions. The good oils are organic flax oil, organic pumpkin seed oil, fresh walnut oil, organic soybean oil, and organic canola oil. Table 18.1 provides a comparison of oils.

Because of food degradation and processing, the amount of intact omega-3 fatty acids in our diet has declined by 80%. The more robust omega-6 fatty acids have survived modern food processing better, so the ratio of omega-6 to omega-3 fatty acids in our diet has increased to about 20:1, instead of the correct ratio it used to

Table 18.1. Colgan Institute Oil Index*

Oil*	Omega-6 Linoleic Acid	Omega-3 Alpha-Linolenic Acid	Monosaturated Fats	Saturated Fats
Good Oils				
Flaxseed (linseed)	14	54	23	9
Pumpkin seed	45	15	32	8
Soybean	44	11	30	15
Walnut	50	5	29	16
Canola	26	8	57	9
Second Best Oils				
Almond	17	—	68	15
Virgin Olive	12	—	72	16
Safflower	70	—	18	12
Sunflower	66	—	22	12
Corn	59	—	25	16
Sesame	42	—	45	13
Rice Bran	35	—	48	17
Bad Oils				
Peanut**	29	—	56	15
Cottonseed***	48	—	28	24
Ugly Oils				
Palm	9	—	44	48
Palm kernel	2	—	18	80
Coconut	4	—	8	88

* Because fat composition of vegetable oils depends somewhat on plant variety and farming methods, some figures have changed from previous tables published by the Colgan Institute. Figures here reflect the latest assays by the major growers.

** Contains carcinogenic aflatoxin

*** May contain toxins.   © Colgan Institute 2006 be, 1:2, before our food supply became degraded by intensive agriculture and processing.[4, 5] The ratio of 20:1 is a certain recipe for disease. Organic flax oil reverses this ratio. It contains only one part omega-6 to four parts omega-3. It contains by far the highest amount of omega-3 fats of any common food. It's inexpensive, too. So flax oil should be your first choice to correct the long-standing omega-3 deficiency prevalent in Western diets. We recommend a tablespoon per day (12–18 grams). Restoration of this balance is especially important in cancer prevention.

Prostaglandins

Prostaglandins are short-lived, hormone-like compounds that your body makes in a series of steps from the two essential fats linoleic acid (omega-6) and alpha-linolenic acid (omega-3). In healthy folk, prostaglandins work in harmony with each other. But for folk deficient in essential fats, they run rampant.

To date, researchers have identified more than 30 different types of prostaglandins. They are grouped in three series according to the fat they are made from. As Figure 18.1 shows, Series 1 and 2 prostaglandins are made from the omega-6 chain. Series 3 are made from the omega-3 chain.

Many prostaglandin functions are still being discovered. Those we know quite a bit about are called E_1, E_2, and E_3. In action, they variously complement or oppose each other. Let's look at these a little closer.

E1: The Protector

Prostaglandin E_1 helps to stop your platelets sticking together to

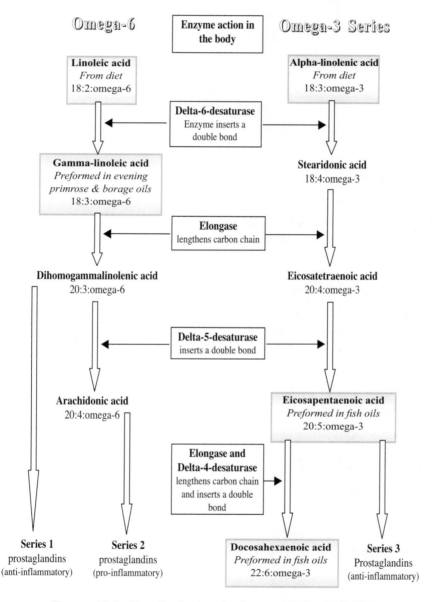

Figure 18.1. How the human body converts essential fats
to fats with special functions.

form clots. It also lowers your blood pressure, inhibits osteoarthritis, reduces pain and inflammatory reactions, and promotes excretion of excess sodium via your kidneys.

E_1 also inhibits release of arachidonic acid from cell membranes where it is stored. As long as it stays in store, arachidonic acid can't be converted to prostaglandin E_2. Thus E_1 prevents excess E_2 production.[6, 7] This is an important function, as we will see.

The bad news is that, even if you do get enough linoleic acid, you still may be unable to produce sufficient prostaglandin E_1. To make E_1, your body has to be able to turn linoleic acid into gamma-linolenic acid. As Figure 18.1 shows, this conversion requires the **delta-6-desaturase** enzyme.

This enzyme function is damaged by a wide variety of stressors. High levels of saturated fats, cholesterol, or trans fats (the bad ones) in your diet, zinc deficiency, excess alcohol consumption, and multiple factors in the degeneration of usual aging all compromise delta-6-desaturase and inhibit production of prostaglandin E_1.[5] And without the protector E_1, prostaglandin E_2 quickly gets out of control.

E2: The Grinch

Prostaglandin E_2 is made from the end fat of the omega-6 chain, arachidonic acid. It promotes platelet clumping, tells your kidneys to retain salt, and increases pain and inflammation. In several ways, it is exactly opposed in action to prostaglandin E_1.

E_2 is necessary to stop bleeding in injuries, to warn you with pain not to exert an injured body part, to promote immune action in infections and illnesses, and to prevent dehydration. But in Western

Society, widespread overproduction of E_2 causes hypertension, sodium and water retention, and chronically inflamed bodies with swollen, painful joints. E_2 needs E_1 to keep it in check.

Prostaglandin E_1 and E_2 are both made from the same essential fat. But the trouble lies in our high red meat consumption. The saturated fats in meat that inhibit delta-6-desaturase are only part of the problem. Even the leanest meat is loaded with preformed arachidonic acid, the direct precursor of E_2. So the saturated fats inhibit the conversion to E_1, and then the meat loads the body with arachidonic acid, thereby boosting production of the pro-inflammatory E_2.[8]

E3: The Defender

As Figure 18.1 shows, your body manufactures E_3 from the next to last step of the omega-3 chain, **eicosapentaenoic acid**. Both eicosapentaenoic acid (EPA) and E_3 prevent production and activity of arachidonic acid even more strongly than E_1. But we have destroyed the alpha-linolenic acid in our food chain to such an extent that 80% of the population is now deficient. Most folk don't get sufficient structural materials to produce enough eicosapentaenoic acid to maintain E_3 production.

As with E_1, saturated fats, trans fats, excess alcohol, and mineral deficiencies in our average diet all inhibit delta-6-desaturase. This important enzyme is needed for the omega-3 chain also.

You can avoid this problem for omega-6 oils by taking pre-formed gamma-linolenic acid. Borage oil, evening primrose oil and blackcurrant oil are all good choices and will help increase your E_1 production. **Wild** coldwater fish (not farmed), such as salmon, mackerel, sardines, and trout, contain good supplies of eicosapentaenoic acid. Or you can use an EPA supplement to boost prostaglandin E_3.

Cancer Prevention

The above biochemistry of essential fats is vital information for cancer prevention. Results from epidemiological studies and experimental studies using animal models indicate that the level of fat in the diet, and more importantly the nature of the constituent fatty acids, influence both breast cancer risk and the progression of the disease.[9] High-fat diets, even if they are rich in omega-6 fatty acids, stimulate breast cancer development and tumor progression. The long-chain omega-3 fatty acids inhibit breast cancer.[9]

Other researchers have established that the omega-6 fatty acid linoleic acid, and in particular arachidonic acid, have a strong growth-promoting effect on many rodent tumors and on human tumor grafts grown in immuno-deficient rodents. By comparison, omega-3 fatty acids are recognized cancer chemopreventive agents.[10]

Many, many studies have now confirmed the anticancer activity of omega-3 fatty acids. In a potent example of the synergistic action of nutrients, one recent representative study showed that omega-3 fatty acids, in combination with antioxidants such as vitamins E and C, increased the anti-cancer effects of both groups of nutrients.[11]

Another recent study, using mice as the experimental model, examined melatonin for its antioxidant activity and flaxseed oil as a source of omega-3 essential fats.[12] The flaxseed oil alone delayed the growth of mammary tumors, only when the omega-6 to omega-

3 ratio was reduced to 1:1. Melatonin on its own delayed the appearance of tumors and slowed tumor growth. The combination of flaxseed oil and melatonin was much more potent. It reduced both the number of tumors and tumor size.[12]

Conjugated linoleic acid (CLA) has caught recent media attention, and some popular press reports cite it as superior fat for health. Don't be fooled. This fatty acid is not an essential fat. It is actually an omega-7 fat [18:2(n-7)] which the body can make. A recent study used the mouse model and induced intestinal tumors to compare anti-tumor activity of fatty acids. In the omega-3 chain, they examined eicosapentaenoic acid, docosahexaenoic acid, alpha-linolenic acid, and stearidonic acid. In the omega-6 chain, they examined gamma-linolenic acid. They also examined conjugated linoleic acid.[13]

Compared with controls, tumor numbers were lower by *half* in those mice fed eicosapentaenoic acid. Docosahexaenoic acid produced only small benefits. Alpha-linolenic acid was ineffective in affecting tumor growth, but it did affect prostaglandin levels. Conjugated linoleic acid (omega-7) and gamma-linolenic acid (omega-6) were ineffective.[13]

From the above and similar evidence, we recommend that you get at least 10 grams per day of omega-3 fatty acids. Your best sources are a tablespoon or two of organic flaxseed oil each day and at least one meal of *wild* cold-water fish, such as steelhead, salmon, mackerel, or sardines, minimally cooked. Wild salmon sashimi is the best fish source. Note well the "wild." Farmed fish, like feedlot beef, grow distorted fats of little value to human health.

An easy way to use flax oil is as salad dressing, mixed to taste with balsamic vinegar and fresh herbs. Cooking destroys essential fats, but they remain undamaged if added to dishes such as pasta sauce after cooking is completed, just before serving. You can also supplement with flax or fish oil capsules. Whatever the way, anoint your inner body with omega-3 oils every day.

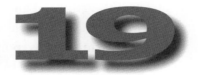

Immunity
Against Cancer

Antioxidants and other vitamins, minerals, and amino acids also prevent cancer by a second mechanism, even more powerful than their direct action to neutralize or prevent the formation of carcinogens. They strengthen and maintain your most important defense against cancer – your immune system. Boosting the immune system not only protects you from cancer, it protects you from everything.

To help you build strong immunity, you need a little information on how it works. The immune system is a body-wide network of specialized cells and processes, roughly divisible into **humoral immunity** and **cell-mediated immunity**. It attacks and usually succeeds in destroying anything that invades your body that it can recognize as alien. That is, substances or organisms which are not a normal part of your structure. Nutrients are not attacked because they occur normally throughout the body.

There are vast armies of aliens. First are all the natural aliens with which we have co-existed throughout our evolution: bacteria and viruses, fungi and molds, poisons from plants, animals and insects, solar radiation, and toxic minerals such as lead and mercury. In the amounts we are usually exposed to, your immune system deals with these invaders very well.

In the last few hundred years, however, we have added tens of thousands of pesticides and herbicides, industrial and medical chemicals, prescription drugs, metal alloys, plastics, gasoline, alien forms of radiation, and superbugs bred by overuse of antibiotics. These unnatural invaders never existed on Earth before. Consequently, your immune system has not had the evolutionary millennia necessary to develop mechanisms to deal with them. Although it tries valiantly, man-made aliens easily overwhelm human immunity.

Carbon monoxide, for example, is a toxic man-made by-product of gasoline use. It did not exist in our evolutionary environment. Every time you smell car exhaust, carbon monoxide is entering your body. Your immune system cannot recognize it and allows the poison to damage, even kill you, without raising a whimper.

All these alien invaders are called **antigens**. On first contact, the humoral division of your immune system tries to make a specific **antibody** for each antigen, capable of recognizing only that one. As you become exposed to more and more antigens, you build a huge library of thousands of different antibodies, a lifelong **immunologic memory** encoded in proteins. With proper maintenance, it protects you very well against the natural aliens, but not so well against man-made aliens.

The cell-mediated division of your immune system is composed of specialized cells, which attack and subdue aliens in microscopic hand-to-hand battles every day. The most important are the **T-cell** and **B-cell lymphocytes**. These are divided into many different subsets with different reactions.   Most lymphocytes use your antibody memory bank to enable them to recognize and attack invading antigens. Whenever they attack, their numbers multiply rapidly. This is called the **lymphocyte proliferative response**. The stronger it is, the stronger your immunity. A look at a few of the main lymphocytes will give you an idea how they work.

Natural killer cells are large lymphocytes that do not need an antibody response in order to recognize some of the aliens. They attack unknown invaders immediately without waiting up to ten days for antibodies to be activated.[1] Natural killer cells are your first line of defense that keeps a new virus or other invader at bay until the antigen-specific immune response can occur.

Phagocytes are the cannibalistic foot soldiers of the immune system. Whenever the body is invaded by foreign or toxic particles, an inflammatory response occurs that brings phagocytes scurrying to the site where they busily ingest dead and dying body cells. They also engulf and kill invading cells, especially if the invaders have already been tagged by antibodies. Your two main phagocytes are called **macrophages** and **neutrophils**. They ingest a wide range of particles from viruses and bacteria to poisons and even tiny fragments of plastic.[2] Eating the aliens kills the phagocytes, too, and the dead cells and their alien contents are then excreted from the body via the bloodstream.

When battling aliens, macrophages, and neutrophils use a lot of oxygen as a weapon. This **oxidative burst** produces a ton of free radicals, which are damaging to the body. The smaller the oxidative burst necessary to destroy invaders, the better your immunity. It is here that antioxidants are so important, both the endogenous ones your body make and those you obtain through your food and supplements. They clean up the free radical mess left by your body's fight with aliens.

Antioxidants to the Rescue

The toxic effects of oxygen radicals produced by your immune cells are controlled to a certain degree by your endogenous antioxidants. But they need the help of nutrient antioxidants to maintain the immune system at its peak. The phagocytes in particular need a mass of antioxidants to support their functions.[3]

Vitamins C and E, for example, are free radical scavengers that improve the immune response.[4] Long-term supplementation with vitamin C definitely reduces the amount of oxygen radicals produced by neutrophils.[5] And diets high in vitamin E improve the action of macrophages and lymphocytes.[6]

Several hundred recent studies have confirmed that antioxidant supplementation improves immune function in the elderly. One representative study investigated vitamins C and E, riboflavin, pyridoxine, iron, and zinc. The researchers concluded that vitamin and mineral intake is an important determinant of immunocompetence.[7] Another recent study examined supplementation with just vitamins C and E. The researchers concluded that these antioxidants are essential for maintenance of immune function in older people and for prevention of heart disease and cancer, the diseases most strongly associated with age.[8]

One of your important endogenous (made by the body) antioxidants is glutathione. Depletion of glutathione is a common consequence of increased formation of free radicals during activity of the immune system. This occurs in the lymphocyte system during development of the immune response and in muscle cells during strenuous exercise.

You can replenish glutathione easily with a protein drink made with 30 grams of whey protein concentrate or isolate.[9] When buying whey concentrates or isolates, look for "ion-exchange" or "cross-flow membrane filtered" forms. Only these products have sufficient pure whey protein to protect you.

Specific Amino Acids Help

Experimental studies show that deficiencies in specific amino acids weaken immunity because they impair antibody synthesis. **L-arginine** is particularly important. Dietary supplementation with this amino acid enhances the cellular immune response of T-lymphocytes. Studies show it also reduces growth of transplantable tumors, lowers the incidence of metastases, and reduces the tumor-producing potential of carcinogens.[10, 11] L-arginine is freely available in the United States, Australia, New Zealand, and recently in Canada. We use 1–3 grams of L-arginine per day.

The amino acid **glutamine** is also vital to immunity. All cell replication in the immune system requires glutamine. Immune cells, however, cannot make glutamine. It is made almost exclusively by your muscle cells. But the immune system uses a ton of it. Your muscles have to supply large amounts of glutamine continuously to your immune system.[12, 13] Anyone with low muscle mass is compromising their immune system.

Unfortunately for your immune system, glutamine is also the main anti-catabolic agent in muscle. This is the compound that helps preserve muscle during and after exercise. So the heavier your training, the heavier the stress on muscles and the greater the muscle need for glutamine. In these cases, unless you supplement with glutamine, both muscle cells and immune cells will be short-changed. With an inadequate glutamine supply, both strength and immunity decline.[12]

Recent studies have shown that supplementing with glutamine is very effective in improving immune responses.[14, 15] Glutamine, however, taken orally has the unfortunate effect of loading your system with ammonia, a by-product of glutamine metabolism that you are better off without. There are several ways to avoid this. If you use l-glutamine supplements, then take them with the same amount of **alpha-glutaric acid (alpha-ketoglutarate)**. This is the ammonia-free carbon skeleton of glutamine that will scavenge excess ammonia.[16]

Another alternative is to use **ornithine alpha-ketoglutarate (OKG)**. Ornithine alpha-ketoglutarate is a known immune system stimulator, probably because oral OKG generates glutamine and arginine. Some research indicates that oral OKG generates more circulating glutamine than oral glutamine itself.[17] So given the choice, take ornithine alpha-ketoglutarate which provides the body with both glutamine and arginine. We have used doses of 2–5 grams per day.

Carotenoids Boost Immunity

We covered the potent effects of carotenoids against cancer in Chapter 17, but want to mention here that they are also intimately involved in supporting your immune system. The US Department of Agriculture (USDA) is among numerous research institutions that conduct specific tests of carotenoids and immunity. In one recent USDA study, researchers put subjects on a low carotenoid diet for three weeks. Their immune function, measured by antigen challenges to samples of whole blood, declined by 25%.

Subjects were then given a mixed cartotenoid supplement for another three weeks. Immune function increased by 37%, including a 20% increase in natural killer cells. Natural killer cells are your first line of defense against alien substances that invade the body.[18]

In previous chapters, we covered the vitamins and carotenoids that support immunity, in addition to their other roles against cancer. There is no need to repeat the amounts we use here. More specific to immunity is the action of whey protein (ion-exchange or cross-flow membrane extraction isolate or concentrate) and the amino acids L-glutamine, L-arginine, and ornithine alpha-ketoglutarate. For these nutrients, the amounts we use are given in Table 19.1 below.

Table 19.1. Nutrients That Maintain Immunity

Nutrient	Daily Amount
Whey protein (isolate or concentrate)	30 grams
L-glutamine with alpha-ketoglutarate	2 – 5 grams
L-arginine with alpha-ketoglutarate **OR**	2 – 5 grams
Ornithine alpha-ketoglutarate	2 – 5 grams

© Colgan Institute 2004

Remember, poor immunity is strongly linked to numerous cancers, as well as arthritis, autoimmune diseases, and increased susceptibility to infectious diseases.[19, 20] Make these nutrients an integral part of your armor.

20

Shining Armor

Since the turn of the millennium, we have started to win the war against cancer. We are not winning with better treatments of established disease, although these have improved. We are winning by prevention of cancer and by prevention and cure of precancerous conditions, such as stomach ulcers, colon disease, and various infections.

Overall cancer death rates are starting to fall in the United States and in Canada, after rising precipitously for most of the 20th century. The Big Four – lung, breast, prostate, and colorectal cancers – remain strong enemies, but are slowly retreating. Now is the time to press our advantage. As people better understand how 80–90% of all cancers are caused by poor nutrition, faulty lifestyle and environmental conditions, tens of thousands are making the personal choices necessary to avoid cancer. Your personal answer to cancer lies in prevention, prevention, prevention. In my case, after 21 years of cancer survival, and for many others like me, it is prevention of recurrence.

Numerous causes of cancer, such as poor nutrition and unprotected sex, are a simple matter of personal choice. Others, like overweight and addiction to smoking, are harder to deal with, but given the strategies herein, still lie within your power to control. Eliminate smoking, and you cut cancer risk by 33%. Maintain a lean body for life, and you cut the risk a further 25%. Just those two cut your overall risk of cancer by 58%.

The next biggest cause of cancer is poor nutrition. I have detailed the strategies to fix it in Chapters 5–7 and 12–18. I have also referred you to my new book, *Nutrition For Champions*, which documents the correct foods to eat to support your genetic design. With the right nutrition, you cut your risk of cancer by another 16%. Now we have removed 74% of all cancer risks.

Cancer-proof your home, avoid cancer in the workplace, and be careful of ultraviolet light, as detailed in Chapters 8 and 9, and you cut cancer risk by another 8%. Avoid excess alcohol and illicit drugs and, as much as possible, prescription drugs, and you cut risk by another 4%. Now we have removed 86% of all cancer risks.

Avoid or control the cancer-causing infections as detailed in Chapter 11 and strengthen your immunity as outlined in Chapter 19. and you cut cancer risk by a further 7%. ***Overall, you have now cut 93% of the risk of all cancers from your life.*** And, in the process, as a bonus, you have cut the risks of many other diseases too. Of the remaining 7%, of cancers, about 2% are genetically caused and 5% are of unknown cause. I'm betting you will have stymied a lot of those as well.

Ninety-three percent is a great bet. I hope this book has convinced you to adopt the armor that presents an impenetrable defense against cancer. As more and more people learn this science, and embrace an anti-cancer lifestyle, I expect to see big reductions in cancer in the next two decades. Please join me in the quest to win this war.

References

Chapter 1: The War on Cancer

1. Colgan M. *Prevent Cancer Now*. San Diego: CI Publications, 1989.

2. Bailar JC, Smith EM. Progress against cancer. *New Engl J Med*, 1986; 314:1226.

3. US National Cancer Institute. www.cancer.gov; accessed 9 June 2006.

4. Davis DL, et al. Decreasing cardiovascular disease and increasing cancer among whites in the U.S. from 1973 through 1987. Good news and bad news. *J Amer Med Assoc*, 1994; 271(6):431-437.

5. Abel U. *Chemotherapy of Advanced Epithelial Cancers*. Stuttgart: Hippocrates Verlag, 1990.

6. Sporn M. The war on cancer. *Lancet* 1996; 347:1377- 1381.

7. Faquet G. *The War on Cancer: An Anatomy of Failure*. New York: Springer, 2005.

8. Annual Report to the Nation on Cancer. *J Nat Cancer Inst*, 5 October 2005.

9. Nordqvist C. *Medical News Today*. 17 May 2006, www.medicalnewstoday.com.

10. American Cancer Society. *Cancer Facts and Figures*. Atlanta: ACS, 2006.

Chapter 2: Prevention, Prevention

1. Lichtenstein P, et al. Environmental and heritable factors in the causation of cancer. *New Engl J Med*, 2000; 343:78-85.

2. Adami H, et al. Primary and secondary prevention in the reduction of cancer morbidity and mortality. *Eur J Cancer*, 2001; Suppl 8:118-127.

3. Hoover RN. Cancer – nature, nurture or both. *New Engl J Med*, 2000; 343, www.nejm.org/content/2000/0343/0002/0135.asp; accessed 22 May 2006

4. Colgan M. *Prevent Cancer Now*. San Diego: CI Publications, 1990.

5. Ames BN, Gold LS. Environmental pollution, pesticides and the prevention of cancer: misconceptions. *FASEB J*, 1997; 11:1041-52.

6. Josefson D. Obesity and inactivity fuel global cancer epidemic. *Brit Med J*, 2001;

322:945.

7.   Montesano R, Hall J. Environmental causes of human cancers. *Eur J Cancer,* 2001; 37, Suppl 8:67-87.

8.   zen Hausen H. Papilloma viruses and cancer. *Nature Reviews,* 2002; 2:342-350.

Chapter 3: No Smoke Without Cancer

1.   Hecht SS. Tobacco and cancer; approaches using carcinogen biomarkers and chemoprevention. *Ann NY Acad Sci,* 1997; 833:91-111.

2.   Johnson BE. Tobacco and lung cancer. *Prim Care,* 1998; 25:279-291.

3.   Hernandez-Boussard TM, Hainaut P. A specific spectrum of p53 mutations in lung cancer from smokers: review of mutations compiled in the IARC p53 database. *Environ Health Perspect,* 1998; 106(7):385-391.

4.   Hackshaw AK. Lung cancer and passive smoking. *Stat Methods Med Res,* 1998; 7:119-136.

5.   Doll R. Uncovering the effects of smoking: historical perspective. *Stat Methods Med Res,* 1998; 7:87-117.

6.   Lewin F, et al. Smoking tobacco, oral snuff, and alcohol in the etiology of squamous cell carcinoma of the head and neck: a population-based case-referent study in Sweden. *Cancer,* 1998; 82(7):1367-1375.

7.   De Stefani E, et al. Tobacco smoking and alcohol drinking as risk factors for stomach cancer: a case-control study in Uruguay. *Cancer Causes Control,* 1998; 9:321-329.

8.   Kanetsky PA, et al. Cigarette smoking and cervical dysplasia among non-Hispanic black women. *Cancer Detect Prev,* 1998; 22:109-119.

9.   Daly SF, et al. Can the number of cigarettes smoked predict high-grade cervical intraepithelial neoplasia among women with mildly abnormal cervical smears? *Amer J Obstet Gynecol,* 1998; 179:399-402.

10.   Ammenheuser MM, et al. Frequencies of hprt mutant lymphocytes in marijuana-smoking mothers and their newborns. *Mutat Res,* 1998; 403:55-64.

11.   Barksky SH, et al. Histopathologic and molecular alterations in bronchial epithelium in habitual smokers of marijuana, cocaine, and/or tobacco. *J Nat Cancer Inst,* 1998; 90:1198-1205.

12.   Hurt RD, Robertson CR. Prying open the door to the tobacco industry's secrets about nicotine. *J Amer Med Assoc,* 1998; 280:1173-1181.

13. Thun MJ, Burns DM. Health Impact of "reduced yield" cigarettes: a critical assessment of the epidemiological evidence. *Tob Control*, 2001; 10(Suppl 1):14-111.

14. Health Canada Tobacco Control Programs. www.hc-sc.ca, January 2004; accessed 20 May 2006.

15. Colgan Institute Anti-aging Seminars. Canada: Saltspring Island, BC, August 2004.

16. American Lung Association. www.lungaction.org/reports/reportcard05; accessed 23 May 2006.

Chapter 4: Overweight Causes Cancer

1. Colgan M. *The New Nutrition: Medicine for the Millenium*. San Diego: CI Publications, 1990.

2. American Cancer Society. *Cancer Prevention Study, 1959-1979*. New York: American Cancer Society, 1980.

3. Schindler AE. Obesity and risk of cancer in the woman. *Zentralbl Gynakol*, 1998; 120:235-40.

4. Chow WH, et al. Body mass index and risk of adenocarcinomas of the esophagus and gastric cardia. *J Nat Cancer Inst*, 1998; 90:150-155.

5. Kaaks R, et al. Breast-cancer incidence in relation to height, weight and body-fat distribution in the Dutch "DOM" cohort. *Int J Cancer*, 1998; 76:647-651.

6. Chang S, et al. Inflammatory breast cancer and body mass index. *J Clin Oncol*, 1998; 16:3731-3735.

7. Zelmanowicz A, et al. Evidence for a common etiology for endometrial carcinomas and malignant mixed mullerian tumors. *Gynecol Oncol*, 1998; 69:253-257.11.

8. Sato F, et al. Body fat distribution and uterine leiomyomas. *J Epidemiol*, 1998; 8:176-180.

9. Weiderpass E, et al. Occurrence, trends and environment etiology of pancreatic cancer. *Scand J Work Environ Health*, 1998; 24:165-174.

10. Silverman DT, et al. Dietary and nutritional factors and pancreatic cancer; a case-control study based on direct interviews. *J Nat Cancer Inst*, 1998; 90:1710-1719.

11. Caan BJ, et al. Body size and the risk of colon cancer in a large case-control study. *Int J Obes Relat Metab Disord*, 1998; 22:178-184.

12. Bird CL, et al. Obesity, weight gain, large weight changes, and adenomatous

polyps of the left colon and rectum. *Amer J Epidemiol*, 1998; 147:670-680.

13.   Cerhan JR, et al. Association of smoking, body mass, and physical activity with risk of prostate cancer in the Iowa 65+ Rural Health Study. *Cancer Causes Control*, 1997; 8:229-238.

14.   Colgan M. *Nutrition For Champions: The 100-Year Diet That Will Keep You Lean For Life*. Vancouver: CI Publications, 2006.

15.   Colgan M. *The New Power Program*. Vancouver: Apple Publishing, 2001.

16.   Colgan M. *Brain Power*. Vancouver: Apple Publishing, 2006.

17.   Colgan M. *Hormonal Health*. Vancouver: Apple Publishing, 1996.

18.   Chen CL, et al. Hormone replacement therapy in relation to breast cancer. *JAMA*, 2002; 287:734-741.

19.   Regelson W, Kalimi M. Dehydroepiandrosterone (DHEA) – the multi-functional steroid. *Ann NY Acad Sci*, 1994; 719: 564-575.

20.   Hulley S, et al. Cardiovascular disease outcomes during 6.8 years of hormone therapy. *JAMA*, 2002; 288:49-57.

21.   Lacey JV, et al. Menopausal hormone replacement therapy and risk of ovarian cancer. *JAMA*, 2002; 288:334-341.

22.   Parl F. *Estrogens, Estrogen Receptors and Breast Cancer*. Amsterdam: IOS Press, 2000.

23.   Gruber CJ, et al. Production and actions of estrogens. *N Engl J Med*, 2002; 346:340-350.

24.   Kirpitchnckov D, et al. Metformin: an update. *Ann Intern Med*, 2002:137:25-33.

25.   Hess AM, Sullivan DL. Metformin for prevention of type 2 diabetes (July/August) *Ann Pharmacother*, 2004, E pub ahead of print, 18 May 2004.

26.   Colgan M. *The New Nutrition: Medicine for the Millenium*. San Diego: CI Publications, 1994.

Chapter 5: Our Food is Degraded

1.   National Research Council. *Recommended Dietary Allowances*, 10th ed. Washington: National Academy Press, 1989.

2.   Harris R, Karmas E (eds). *Nutritional Evaluation of Food Processing*, 2nd ed. Westport CT: Avi Publishing, 1975.

3. Colgan M. *The New Nutrition: Medicine for the Millenium.* Vancouver: Apple Publishing, 1995.

4. US Dept Agriculture. 1994-1996 Continuing Survey of Food Intakes by Individuals. www.barc.usda.gov/bhnrc/foodsurvey/; accessed 24 May 2006

5. Consumer Reports 2002-2006. www.eco-label.org; accessed 24 May 2006.

6. Environmental Protection Agency. *Report on the Status of Chemicals in the Special Review Program.* Office of Pesticide Programs (TS 767C). Washington: EPA, 1987.

7. Tao SS, Bolger PM. Dietary arsenic intakes in the United States: FDA Total Diet Study, September 1991 – December 1996. *Food Addit Contam*, 1999; 16(11):465-472.

8. Dougherty CP, et al. Dietary exposures to food contaminants across the United States. *Environ Res*, 2000; 84(2):170-185.

9. Schreinemachers DM. Cancer mortality in four northern wheat-producing states. *Environ Health Perspect*, 2000; 108(9):873-881.

10. Ji BT, et al. Occupational exposure to pesticides and pancreatic cancer. *Amer J Ind Med*, 2001; 39(1):92-99.

11. Valdez Salas B, et al. Impact of pesticide use on human health in Mexico: a review. *Rev Environ Health*, 2000; 15(4):399-412.

Chapter 6: Refined Foods Promote Cancer

1. Colgan M. *The New Nutrition: Medicine for the Millennium.* Vancouver: Apple Publishing, 1994.

2. Colgan M. *Optimum Sports Nutrition.* New York: Advanced Research Press, 1993.

3. Colgan M. *Sports Nutrition Guide.* Vancouver: Apple Publishing, 2002.

4. Williams RJ. In Hawkins D, Pauling L. (eds). *Orthomolecular Psychiatry.* San Francisco: WH Freeman, 1973, 316.

5. Williams RJ, Pelton RB. *Proc Nat Acad Sci USA*, 1966; 55:126.

6. Jacobs DR Jr, et al. Is whole grain intake associated with reduced total and cause-specific death rates in older women? The Iowa Women's Health Study. *Amer J Public Health*, 199; 89:322-329.

7. Levi F, et al. Food groups and colorectal cancer risk. *Brit J Cancer,* 1999; 79:1283-1287.

8.   Salmeron J, et al. Dietary fiber, glycemic load, and risk of NIDDM in men. *Diabetes Care*, 1997; 20:545-550.

9.   Boutron-Ruault MC, et al. Foods as risk factors for colorectal cancer: a case-control study in Burgundy (France). *Eur J Cancer Prev*, 1999; 8:229-35.

Chapter 7: Toxic Water Everywhere

1.   Ballester F, Sunyer J. Drinking water and gastrointestinal disease: need of better understanding and an improvement in public health surveillance. *J Epidemiol Comm Health*, 2000; 54:3-5.

2.   World Health Organization. *Life in the 21ˢᵗ Century. A Vision for All.* The World Health Report 1998. Geneva: WHO, 1998.

3.   MacKenzie W, et al. A massive outbreak in Milwaukee of cryptosporidium infection transmitted through the public water supply. *New Engl J Med*, 1994; 331:161-167.

4.   Ford T. Microbial safety of drinking water: United States and global perspectives. *Environ Health Perspect*, 1999; 107(S1):191-206.

5.   Rose J, et al. Risk assessment and control of waterborne Giardiasis. *Amer J Public Health*, 1991; 81:709-713.

6.   US Dept of Health and Human Servises, CDC. Assessing the public health threat associated with waterborne Cryptosporidiosis: report of a workshop. *Morb Mortal Wkly Rep*, 1995; 44(RR6):1-19.

7.   Payment P, Siemiatycki J, Richardson L, et al. A prospective epidemiological study of gastrointestinal health effects due to the consumption of drinking water. *Int J Environ Health Res*, 1997; 7:5-31.

8.   Payment P, et al. A randomized trial to evaluate the risk of gastrointestinal disease due to consumption of drinking water meeting current microbiological standards. *Amer J Public Health*, 1991; 81:703-708.

9.   Aramini J, et al. Drinking water quality and health-care utilization for gastrointestinal illness in greater Vancouver. *Can Comm Disease Rep*, 2000; 26(24):211-214.

10.   Koivusalo M, Vartiainen T. Drinking water chlorination by-products and cancer. *Rev Environ Health*, 1997; 12(2):81-90.

11.   Bull RJ, et al. Water chlorination: essential process or cancer hazard? *Fundam Appl Toxicol*, 1995; 28(2):155-166.

12. Wigle DT. Safe drinking water: a public health challenge. *Chronic Disease Can,* 1998; 19(3):103-107.

13. Cantor KP. Invited commentary: arsenic and cancer of the urinary tract. *Amer J Epidemiol,* 2001; 153(5):422-423.

14. Yu RC, et al. Arsenic methylation capacity and skin cancer. *Cancer Epidemiol Biomarkers Prev,* 2000; 9(11):1259-1262.

15. Cantor KP, Weissman JD. *Choose to Live.* New York: Penquin Books, 1988.

16. Underwood EJ. *Trace Elements in Human and Animal Nutrition,* 4th ed. New York: Academic Press, 1977:466.

Chapter 8: Cancer at Home and Work

1. Morgan KT. A brief review of formaldehyde carcinogenesis in relation to rat nasal pathology and human health risk assessment. *Toxicol Pathol,* 1997;25(3):291-307.

2. California Environmental Protection Agency. *Formaldehyde in the Home.* Sacramento: California Air Resources Board, August 2004.

3. Ayotte P, et al. Indoor exposure to 222Rn: a public health perspective. *Health Phys,* 1998;75(3):297-302.

4. Wang Y, et al. Radon mitigation survey among New York State residents living in high radon homes. *Health Phys,* 1999,77(4):403-409.

5. US Environmental Protection Agency. Exposure to radon causes lung cancer in smokers and non-smokers alike. www.epa.gov/radon; accessed 9 June 2006.

6. Zahm SH, Ward MH. Pesticides and childhood cancer. *Environ Health Perspect,* 1998;106(S3):893-908.

7. Meinert R, et al. Leukemia and non-Hodgkin's lymphoma in childhood and exposure to pesticides: results of a register-based case-control study in Germany. *Amer J Epidemiol,* 2000;151(7):639-646.

8. Budkley JD, et al. Pesticide exposure in children with non-Hodgkin lymphoma. *Cancer,* 2000;89(11):2315-2321.

9. Bukowski JA, et al. Environmental causes for sinonasal cancers in pet dogs, and their usefulness as sentinels of indoor cancer risk. *J Toxicol Environ Health,* 1998;54(7):579-591.

10. Hayes HM, et al. Case-control study of canine malignant lymphoma: positive association with dog owner's use of 2,4-dichlorophenoxyacetic acid herbicides. *J*

Natl Cancer Inst, 1991;83(17):1226-1231.

11.   Anderson A, et al. Work-related cancers in Nordic countries. *Scand J Work Environ Health*, 1999; 25 Suppl 2: 1-116.

12.   Renner R. Harmful farming. *Environ Health Perspec*, 2002: 110: 445-456.

Chapter 9: Ultra-Violet Causes Cancer

1.   Centers for Disease Control. Cancer Prevention and Control. www.cdc.gov; accessed 24 May 2006.

2.   Autier P, et al. Sunscreen use and the number of nevi in 6-7-year-old European children. *J Nat Cancer Inst*, 1998; 90: 1873-1880.

3.   Veirod MB, et al. A prospective study of pigmentation, sun exposure, and cutaneous malignant melanoma in women. *J Nat Cancer Inst*, 2003; 95: 1530-1538.

4.   Nguyen HL. Melanoma. In Bishop JF (ed), *Cancer Facts: A Concise Oncology Text*. Amsterdam: Harwood Academic Publishers, 1999: 255-259.

5.   Reuters News. UK male deaths from melanoma rising fast. 15 May 2006.

6.   Cokkinides VE, et al. Sun exposure and sun-protection behaviors and attitudes among U.S. youth, 11 to 18 years of age. *Prev Med*, 2001; 33: 141-151.

7.   The Cancer Council: South Australia. Teenagers resist the urge to tan. News release, 14 November 2005.

Chapter 10: Alcohol Promotes Cancer

1.   Ringborg U. Alcohol and risk of cancer. *Alcohol Clin Exp Res*, 1998; 22:323S-328S.

2.   National Research Council. *Diet, Nutrition and Cancer.* Washington: National Academy Press, 1982:5-20.

3.   Seitz HK, et al. Alcohol and cancer. *Recent Dev Alcohol*, 1998; 14:67-95.

4.   Yokoyama A, et al. Alcohol-related cancers and aldehyde dehydrogenase-2 in Japanese alcoholics. *Carcinogenesis*, 1998; 19:1383-1387.

5.   Editorial. Screening for alcoholism. *Lancet*, 1980; 2:1117.

6.   Harvard Medical School. *The Harvard Medical School Health Letter*, 1981; 7:2.

7.   Gronbaek M, et al. Population based cohort study of the association between

alcohol intake and cancer of the upper digestive tract. *Brit Med J*, 1998; 317:844-847.

8.   Berger J. Is silymarin hepato-protective? *J Clin Gastroenterol*, 2003; 37:278-279.

Chapter 11: Infections Cause Cancer

1.   Colgan M. *Prevent Cancer Now*. San Diego: CI Publications 1990.

2.   zur Hausenh H. Papilloma viruses and cancer. *Nature Reviews*, 2002; 2: 342-350.

3.   International Agency for Research on Cancer. Infection with schistosomes. *IARC*, 1994; 61: 45.

4.   Watanapa P. Liver fluke-associated cholangiocarcinoma. *Brit J Surg*, 2002; 89: 962-970.

5.   Dart H. Infections and cancer risk. Harvard Center for Cancer Prevention, www.hsph.harvard.edu/cancer/risk; accessed 25 May 2006.

6.   National Cancer Institute. Gastric cancer. 11 March 2005. http://cancer.gov.

7.   Shehan P. Headline News. Upcoming trial of potential hepatitis C vaccine. 8 May 2006.

8.   Munoz N, et al. The causative link between human papilloma virus and cervical cancer. *Int J Cancer*, 1992; 52: 743-749.

9.   Plescia CJ, et al. AN analytical overview of the microbicide preclinical and clinical pipeline. Microbicides 2006 Conference. Cape Town, South Africa 23-26 April 2006.

10.   Maugh TH. Cervical cancer vaccine one step from approval. *Los Angeles Times*, 19 May 2006.

11.   Lowy DR, Schiller JT. Prophylactic human papilloma virus vaccines. *J Clin Invest*, 2006; 116: 1167-1173..

12.   Epstein MA, et al. Morphological and biological studies on a virus in cultured lymphoblasts from Burkitt's lymphoma. *J Exper Med*, 1965; 121: 761-770.

Chapter 12: Low-Fat Diet Prevents Cancer

1.   The morality of fat. *New York Times*, Fitness and Nutrition, 25 May 2006.

2.   Kim DY, et al. Stimulatory effects of high-fat diets on colon cell proliferation depend on the type of dietary fat and site of the colon. *Nutr Cancer*, 1998; 30:118-123.

3.   Snyderwine EG, et al.   Mammary gland carcinogenicity of 2-amino-1-methyl-6-phenylimidazo [4,5-b]pyridine in Sprague-Dawley rats on high- and low-fat diets. *Nutr Cancer*, 1998; 31:160-167.

4.   National Academy of Sciences. *Diet, Nutrition and Cancer*. Washington, DC: National Academy Press, 1982:5-20.

5.   Hill MJ. Nutrition and human cancer. *Ann NY Acad Sci*, 1997; 833:68-78.

6.   Snyderwine EG. Diet and mammary gland carcinogenesis. *Recent Results Cancer Res*, 1998; 152:3-10.

7.   Boyd NF, et al.   Effects at two years of a low-fat, high-carbohydrate diet on radiologic features of the breast: results from a randomized trial.   Canadian Diet and Breast Cancer Prevention Study Group. *J Nat Cancer Inst*, 1997; 89:488-496.

8.   Boyd NF, et al.   Effects of a low-fat high-carbohydrate diet on plasma sex hormones in premenopausal women: results from a randomized controlled trial. Canadian Diet and Breast Cancer Prevention Study Group. *Brit J Cancer*, 1997; 76:127-135.

9.   Colgan M. *Protect Your Prostate*. Vancouver: Apple Publishing, 2000.

10.   Xue L, et al. Induced hyperproliferation in epithelial cells of mouse prostate by a Western-style diet. *Carcinogenesis*, 1997; 18:995-999.

11.   Whittemore AS, et al.   Prostate cancer in relation to diet, physical activity and body size in blacks, whites and Asians in the United States and Canada. *J Nat Cancer Inst*, 1995; 87:652-661.

12.   Bairati I, et al. Dietary fat and advanced prostate cancer. *J Urol*, 1998; 159:1271-1275.

13.   American Prostate Society. Update. Summer/Fall, 1997:1.

14.   Colgan M. *Essential Fats*. Vancouver: Apple Publishing, in press.

Chapter 13: Fiber Prevents Cancer

1.   American Cancer Society. *Cancer Facts and Figures*. Atlanta: ACS 2006

2.   Liu K, et al. Dietary cholesterol, fat, and fibre, and colon-cancer mortality. An analysis of international data. *Lancet*, 1979; 2:782-785.

3.   Maclennan R, et al. Dietary fibre, transit-time, faecal bacteria, steroids, and colon cancer in two Scandinavian populations. *Lancet*, 1977; 2:207-211.

4.   Story JA, Kritchevsky D. Comparison of the binding of various bile acids and

bile salts in vitro by several types of fiber. *J Nutr*, 1976; 106:1292-1294.

5. Reddy BS, Wynder EL. Large-bowel carcinogenesis: fecal constituents of populations with diverse incidence rates of colon cancer. *J Nat Cancer Inst*, 1973; 50:1437-1442.

6. Burkitt DP. Effect of dietary fibre on stools and the transit-times, and its role in the causation of disease. *Lancet,* 1972; 2:1408-1412.

7. DeCosse JJ, et al. Effect of wheat fiber and vitamins C and E on rectal polyps in patients with familial adenomatous polyposis. *J Nat Cancer Inst*, 1989; 81:1290-1297.

8. Jansen MC, et al. Dietary fiber and plant foods in relation to colorectal cancer mortality: the Seven Countries Study. *Int J Cancer*, 1999; 81:174-179.

9. National Cancer Institute. *Cancer Prevention.* HIH Publication No. 84-2671. Washington: Department of Health and Human Services, 1984.

10. Colgan M. *Nutrition For Champions: The 100-Year Diet That Will Keep You Lean For Life.* Vancouver: Apple Publishing, 2006.

Chapter 14: Vitamins and Cancer

1. Schorah CJ. Micronutrients, antioxidants and risk of cancer. *Bibl Nutr Dieta*, 1995; (52):92-107.

2. Greenwald P, et al. New directions in dietary studies in cancer: the National Cancer Institute. *Adv Exp Med Biol*, 1995; 369:229-239.

3. Kelloff GJ, et al. Progress in cancer Chemoprevention: development of diet-derived chemopreventive agents. *J Nutr*, 2000; 130(2S):467S-471S.

4. Fletcher RH, Fairfield K. A multivitamin /mineral per day. *J Amer Med Assoc*, 2002; 207: 3127-3129.

5. Patterson BH, et al. Fruit and vegetables in the American diet: data from the NHANES II survey. *Amer J Public Health*, 1990; 80(12):1443-1449.

6. Breslow RA, et al. Trends in food intake: the 1987 and 1992 National Health Interview Surveys. *Nutr Cancer,* 1997:28(1):86-92.

7. Ames BN. Micronutrients prevent cancer and delay aging. *Ann NY Acad Sci*, 1999; 889:87-106.

8. Briefel RR, et al. Zinc intake of the U.S. population: findings from the third National Health and Nutrition Examination Survey, 1988-1994. *J Nutr*, 2000; 130:1367S-1373S.

9.   Block G. Dietary guidelines and their results of food consumption surveys. *Amer J Clin Nutr*, 1991; 53:356S-357S.

10. Colgan M. *Nutrition For Champions: The 100-Year Diet That Will Keep You Lean For Life*. Vancouver: Apple Publishing, 2006.

11. National Research Council. *Recommended Dietary Allowances*, 10th ed. Washington DC: National Academy Press, 1989.

12. Kumpulainen JT. Chromium content of foods and diets. *Biol Trace Elem Res*, 1992; 32:9-18.

13. Hallfrisch J, Muller DC. Does diet provide adequate amounts of calcium, iron, magnesium, and zinc in a well-educated adult population? *Exp Gerontol*, 1993; 28:473-483.

14. Burkitt D, Trowell HC. *Western Diseases: Their Emergence and Prevention*. Cambridge MA: Harvard University Press, 1981.

15. Colgan M. *The New Nutrition: Medicine for the Millenium*. Vancouver: Apple Publishing, 1994.

16. Reddy MB, Love M. The impact of food processing on the nutritional quality of vitamins and minerals. *Adv Exp Med Biol*, 1999; 459:99-106.

17. American Medical Association Council of Food and Nutrition. *Nutrients in Processed Foods*. Acton, MA: Publishing Sciences Group, 1974.

18. Schroeder HA. Losses of vitamins and trace minerals resulting from processing and preservation of foods. *Amer J Clin Nutr*, 1971; 24:562-573.

19. Colgan M. *Optimum Sports Nutrition*. New York: Advanced Research Press, 1993.

20. Colgan M. *Hormonal Health*. Vancouver: Apple Publishing, 1996.

21. Colgan M. *Sports Nutrition Guide*. Vancouver, Apple Publishing, 2002.

Chapter 15: Antioxidants Prevent Cancer

1.   Geruth A, et al. (eds). *Oxy-radicals in Molecular Biology and Pathology*. New York: AR Liss, 1988.

2.   Bartlet N (ed). *The Oxidation of Oxygen and Related Chemistry*. London: World Scientific Publishing, 2001.

3.   Maxiere S, et al. Effect of resistant starch and/or fat-soluble vitamins A nd E on the initiation stage of aberrant cypts in rat colon. *Nutr Cancer*, 1998; 31:168-77.

4. Bojkova B, et al. Effects of retinyl acetate and melatonin on N-methyl-N-nirosouurea-induced mammary carcinogenesis in rats. A preliminary report. *Folia Biol*, 2000; 46:73-76.

5. Ahlersova E, et al. Melatonin and retinyl acetate as chemopreventives in DMBA-induced mammary carcinogenesis in female Sprague-Dawley rats. *Folia Biol*, 2000; 46:69-72.

6. Cameron E, Pauling L. *Cancer and Vitamin C*. New York: Warner Books, 1981.

7. Ames B. *Science*, 1983; 221:1256.

8. Head KA. Ascorbic acid in the prevention and treatment of cancer. *Altern Med Rev*, 1998; 3:174-186.

9. Venugopal M, et al. Synergistic anti-tumour activity of vitamins C and K3 against human prostate carcinoma cell lines. *Cell Biol Int*, 1996; 20:787-797.

10. Schorah CJ. Ascorbic acid metabolism and cancer in the human stomach. *Acta Gastroenterol Belg*, 1997; 60:217-219.

11. Wagner D. *Cancer Res*, 1985; 45:6519.

12. Tavares DC, et al. Protective effects of the amino acid glutamine and of ascorbic acid against chromosomal damage induced by doxorubicin in mammalian cells. *Teratog Carcinog Mutagen*, 1998; 18:153-161.

13. Cameron E, Pauling L. *Cancer and Vitamin C*. California: The Linnus Pauling Institute, 1979.

14. Kneckt P, et al. Vitamin E and cancer prevention. *Am J Clin Nutr*, 1991; 53:283S-286S.

15. Heinonen OP, et al. Prostate cancer and supplementation with alpha-tocopherol and beta-carotene: incidence and mortality in a controlled trial. *J Nat Cancer Inst*, 1998; 90:440-446.

16. McVean M, Liebler DC. Prevention of DNA photodamage by vitamin E compounds and sunscreens: roles of ultraviolet absorbance and cellular uptake. *Mol Carcinog*, 1999; 24:169-176.

17. Clapper ML, Szarka CE. Glutathione S-transferases-biomarkers of cancer risk and chemopreventive response. *Chem Biol Interact*, 1998; 111-112:337-388.

18. Exner R, et al. Therapeutic potential of glutathione. *Wein Klin Wochenschr*, 2000; 112:610-616.

19. Combs GF, Gray WP. Chemopreventive agents: selenium. *Pharmacol Ter*, 1998; 79:179-92.

20. Irion CW. Growing alliums and brassicas in selenium-enriched soils increases their anticarcinogenic potentials. *Med Hypotheses,* 1999; 53:232-235.

21. Jiang C, et al. Selenium-induced inhibition of angiogenesis in mammary cancer at chemopreventive levels of intake. *Mol Carcinog,* 1999; 26:213-225.

22. Yan L, et al. Dietary supplementation of selenomethionine reduces metastasis of melanoma cells in mice. *Anticancer Res,* 1999; 19:1337-1342.

23. Colgan M. *Protect Your Prostate.* Vancouver: Apple Publishing, 2000.

24. Schrauzer GN. Selenium. Mechanistic aspects of anticarcinogenic action. *Biol Trace Elem Res,* 1992; 33:51-62.

25. Colgan M. Trace elements. *Science,* 1981; 124: 744.

26. Hodges S, et al. CoQ10: could it have a role in cancer management? *Biofactors,* 1999; 9:365-370.

27. Matthews RT, et al. Coenzyme Q10 administration increases brain mitochondrial concentrations and exerts neuroprotective effects. *Proc Nat Acad Sci USA,* 1998; 95:8892-8897.

28. Colgan M. *Hormonal Health.* Vancouver, Apple Publishing, 1996.

29. Reiter RJ, et al. a review of the evidence supporting melatonin's role as an antioxidant. *J Pineal Res,* 1995; 18:1-11.

30. Anisimov VN, et al. Melatonin and colon carcinogenesis: I. Inhibitory effect of melatonin on development of intestinal tumors induced by 1,2-dimethylhydrazine in rats. *Carcinogenesis,* 1997; 18:1549-1553.

31. Qi W, et al. Inhibitory effects of melatonin on ferric nitrilotriacetate-induced lipid peroxidation and oxidative DNA damage in the rat kidney. *Toxicology,* 1999; 139:81-91.

32. de Grey AD. *The Mitochondrial Free Radical Theory of Aging.* Georgetown TX: Landes Bioscience, 1999.

33. Harmon D. *J Am Geriat Soc,* 1972; 20:145-147.

34. Colgan M. *Brain Power.* Vancouver: Apple Publishing, 2006.

35. Liu J, et al. Delaying brain mitochondrial decay and aging with mitochondrial antioxidants and metabolites. *Ann NY Acad Sci,* 2002; 959:133-166.

36. Hagen TM, et al. Feeding acetyl-l-carnitine and lipoic acid to old rats significantly improves metabolic functions while decreasing oxidative stress. *Proc Natl Acad Sci,* 2002; 99:1870-1875.

37. Adibharla RM, et al. Citicholine: neuroprotective mechanisms in cerebral

ischemia. *Neurochem*, 2002; 80:12-23.

Chapter 16: Flavonoids Prevent Cancer

1.   Wattenberg LW. In Arnott MS, et al (eds), *Molecular Interactions of Nutrition and Cancer*. New York: Raven Press, 1982:43.

2.   National Academy of Sciences. *Diet, Nutrition and Cancer*. Washington: National Academy Press, 1982:5-20.

3.   Kaul A, Khanduja KL. Polyphenols inhibit promotional phase of tumorigenesis: relevance of superoxide radicals. *Nutr Cancer*, 1998; 32:81-5.

4.   Kuroda Y, Hara Y. Anti-mutagenic and anti-carcinogenic activity of tea polyphenols. *Mutat Res*, 1999; 436:69-97.

5.   Nakachi K, et al. Influence of drinking green tea on breast cancer malignancy among Japanese patients. *Jpn J Cancer Res*, 1998,89:254-261.

6.   Wang ZY, et al. Inhibition of N-nitrosomethylbenzylamine-induced esophageal turmoigenesis in rats by green and black tea. *Carcinogenesis*, 1995; 16:2143-2148.

7.   Mohan RR, et al. Over expression of ornithine decarboxylase in prostate cancer and prostatic fluid in humans. *Clin Cancer Res*, 1999; 5:143-147.

8.   Gupta S, et al. Prostate cancer chemoprevention by green tea: in vitro and in vivo inhibition of testosterone-mediated induction of ornithine decarboxylase. *Cancer Res*, 1999; 59:2115-2120.

9.   Katiyar SK, et al. Protection against induction of mouse skin papillomas with low and high risk of conversion to malignancy by green tea polyphenols. *Carcinogenesis*, 1997; 18:497-502.

10.   Bomser JA, et al. Inhibition of TPA-induced tumor promotion in CD-1 mouse epidermis by a polyphenolic fraction from grape seeds. *Cancer Lett*, 1999; 135:151-157.

11.   Elattar TM, Virji AS. Modulating effect of resveratrol and quercetin on oral cancer cell growth and proliferation. *Anticancer Drugs*, 1999; 10:187-193.

12.   Wong GY, et al. Dose-ranging study of indole-3-carbinol for breast cancer prevention. *J Cell Biochem Suppl*, 1997; 28-29:111-116.

13.   Cover CM, et al. Indole-3-carbinol and tamoxifen cooperate to arrest the cell cycle of MCF-7 human breast cancer cells. *Cancer Res*, 1999, 59:1244-1251.

14.   Manson MM, et al. Chemoprevention of aflatoxin B1-induced carcinogenesis by

indoe-3-carbinol in rate liver – predicting the outcome using early biomarkers. *Carcinogenesis*, 1998; 19:1829-1836.

15. Xu X, et al. Effects of soy isoflavones on estrogen and phytoestrogen metabolism in premenopausal women. *Cancer Epidemiol Biomarkers Prev*, 1998; 7:1101-1108.

16. Zheng W, et al. Urinary excretion of isoflavonoids and the risk of breast cancer. *Cancer Epidemiol Biomarkers Prev*, 1999; 8:35-40.

17. Katdare M, et al. Inhibition of aberrant proliferation and induction of apoptosis in preneoplastic human mammary epithelial cells by natural phytochemicals. *Oncol Rep*, 1998; 5:311-315.

18. Davis JN, et al. Genistein-induced up-regulation of p21WAF1, down-regulation of cyclin B, and induction of apoptosis in prostate cancer cells. *Nutr Cancer*, 1998; 32:123-131.

19. Zhou, JR, et al. Inhibition of murine bladder tumorigenesis by soy isoflavones via alterations in the cell cycle, apoptosis and angiogenesis. *Cancer Res*, 1998; 58:5231-5238.

20. Lian F, et al. Genistein-induced G2-M arrest, p21WAF1 up-regulation, and apoptosis in a non-small-cell lung cancer cell line. *Nutr Cancer*, 1998; 31:184-191.

21. Inano H, et al. Chemoprevention by curcumin during the promotion stage of tumorigenesis of mammary gland in rats irradiated with gamma-rays. *Carcinogenesis*, 1999; 20:1011-1018.

22. Kawamori T, et al. Chemopreventive effect of curcumin, a naturally occurring anti-inflammatory agent, during the promotion/progression stages of colon cancer. *Cancer Res*, 1999; 59:597-601.

23. Zhang Y, Talalay P. Mechanism of differential potencies of isothiocyanates as inducers of anti-carcinogenic Phase 2 enzymes. *Cancer Res*, 1998; 58:4632-4639.

24. Shapiro TA, et al. Human metabolism and excretion of cancer chemoprotective glucosinolates and isothiocyanates of cruciferous vegetables. *Cancer Epidemiol Biomarkers Prev*, 1998; 7:1091-1100.

25. Hecht SS. Chemoprevention of cancer by isothiocyantes, modifiers of carcinogen metabolism. *J Nutr*, 1999; 129:768S-774S.

26. Stoner GD, et al. Inhibition of N'-nitrosonornicotine-induced esophageal tumorigenesis by 3-phenylpropyl isothiocyanate. *Carcinogenesis*, 1998; 19:2139-2143.

Chapter 17: Carotenoids Prevent Cancer

1. Ben-Amotz A, Levy Y. Bioavailability of a natural isomer mixture compared with synthetic all-trans beta-carotene in human serum. *Am J Clin Nutr*, 1996:63:729-734.

2. Bendich A, Butterworth CE (eds). *Micronutrients in Health and Disease.* Marcel Dekker, 1991.

3. Smith W, et al. Dietary antioxidants and age-related maculopathy. *Opthalmology*, 1999:106:761-767.

4. Freudenheim JL, et al. Premenopausal breast cancer risk and intake of vegetables, fruits and related nutrients. *J Natl Cancer Inst*, 1966; 88:340-348.

5. Zhang S, et al. Dietary carotenoids and vitamins A, C and E and risk of breast cancer. *J Nat Cancer Inst*, 1999; 91:547-556.

6. Batieha AM, et al. Serum micronutrients and the subsequent risk of cervical caner in a population-based nested case-control study. *Cancer Epidemiol Biomark Prev*, 1993; 2:335-339.

7. Barbone F, et al. A follow-up study of determinants of second tumor and metastasis among subjects with cancer of the oral cavity, pharynx and larynx. *J Clin Epidemiol*, 1996; 49:367-372.

8. Franceschi S, et al. Tomatoes and risk of digestive tract cancers. *Int J Cancer*, 1994; 59:181-184.

9. Nomura AM, et al. Serum vitamin levels and risk of cancer of specific sites in men of Japanese ancestry in Hawaii. *Cancer Res*, 1985; 45:2369-2372.

10. Ziegler RG, et al. Importance of alpha-carotene, beta-carotene and other phytochemicals in the etiology of lung cancer. *J Nat Cancer Inst*, 1996; 88:612-615.

11. Giovanucci E, et al. Intake of carotenoids and retinol in relation to risk of prostate cancer. *J Natl Cancer Inst*, 1995; 87:1767-1776.

Chapter 18: Essential Fats Prevent Cancer

1. Colgan M. *Your Personal Vitamin Profile.* New York: William Morrow, 1982.

2. Horrobin DF. Essential Fatty Acids: A Review. In Horrobin DF (ed), *Clinical Use of Fatty Acids.* London: Eden Press, 1982.

3. National Academy of Sciences. *Recommended Dietary Allowances*, 10th ed. National Academy Press, 1989.

4.   Kabara J. *Pharmacological Effects of Lipids*, Vol I, II, III. Champaign, IL: ACOS, 1978, 1985, 1989.

5.   Erasmus U. *Fats That Heal: Fats That Kill*, 2nd ed. Burnaby: Alive Books, 1993.

6.   Brisson GJ. *Lipids in Human Nutrition*. New York, NY: Burgess, 1981.

7.   Willis A. Handbook of Eicosanoids, *Prostaglandins & Related Lipids*, Vol 1 & 2. Boca Raton, FL: CRC Press, 1987, 1989.

8.   Colgan M. *Essential Fats*. Vancouver: Apple Publishing, in press.

9.   Rose DP. Dietary fats, fatty acids and breast cancer. *Breast Cancer*, 1997; 4:7-16.

10.   Sauer LA, et al. Mechanism for the antitumor and anticachectic effects of n-3 fatty acids. *Cancer Res*, 2000; 60:5289-5295.

11.   Yam D, et al. Suppression of tumor growth and metastasis by dietary fis oil combined with vitamins E and C and cisplatin. *Cancer Chemother Pharmacol*, 2001; 47:34-40.

12.   Rao GN, et al. Effect of melatonin and linolenic acid on mammary cancer in transgenic mice with c-neu breast cancer oncogene. *Breast Cancer Res Treat*, 2000; 64:287-296.

13.   Petrik MB, et al. Highly unsaturated (n-3) fatty acids, but not alpha-linolenic, conjugated linoleic or gamma-linolenic acids, reduce tumorigenesis in Apc(Min/+) mice. *J Nutr*, 2000; 130:2434-2443.

Chapter 19: Immunity Against Cancer

1.   Herberman RB, Ortaldo JR. Natural killer cells: their role in defenses against disease. *Science*, 1981; 214:24-30.

2.   Golub ES, Green DR. *Immunology: A Synthesis*. 2nd ed. Sunderland, MA: Sinauer, 1991.

3.   Del Rio M, et al. Improvement by several antioxidants of macrophage function in vitro. *Life Sci*, 1998; 63:871-881.

4.   Victor VV, et al. Ascorbic acid modulates in vitro the function of macrophages from mice with endotoxic shock. *Immunopharmacology*, 2000; 46:89-101.

5.   Ellis GR, et al. Neutrophil superoxide anion-generating capacity, endothelial function and oxidative stress in chronic heart failure: effects of short- and long-term vitamin C therapy. *J Amer Coll Cardiol*, 1000; 35:1474-1482.

6.   De la Fuente M, et al. Changes in macrophage and lymphocyte functions in

guinea-pigs after different amounts of vitamin E ingestion. *Brit J Nutr*, 2000; 84:25-29.

7. Buzina-Suboticanec K, et al. Aging, nutritional status and immune response. *Int J Vitam Nutr Res*, 1998; 68:133-141.

8. De la Fuente M, et al. Immune function in aged women is improved by ingestion of vitamins C and E. *Can J Physiol Pharmacol*, 1998; 76:373-380.

9. Bounous G. Whey protein concentrate (WPC) and glutathione modulation in cancer treatment. *Anticancer Res*, 2000; 20:4785-4792.

10. Ochoa JB, et al. Effects of L-arginine on the proliferation of T lymphocyte subpopulations. *J Parenter Enteral Nutr*, 2001; 25:23-29.

11. Novaes MR, Lima LA. Effects of dietetic supplementation with L-arginine in cancer patients. A review of the literature. *Arch Latinoam Nutr*, 1999; 49:301-308.

12. Newsholme EA. Psychoimmunology and cellular nutrition: an alternative hypothesis. *Biol Psychiat*, 1990; 27:1-3.

13. Griffiths M, Keast D. The effect of glutamine on murine splenic leucocyte responses to T- and B-cell mitogens. *Cell Biology*, 1990; 68:405-408.

14. Field CJ, et al. Glutamine and arginine: immunonutrients for improved health. *Med Sci Sports Exerc*, 2000; 32:S377-388.

15. Calder PC, Yaqoob P. Glutamine and the immune system. *Amino Acids*, 1999; 17:227-241.

16. Wernerman J, et al. Alpha-ketoglutarate and postoperative muscle catabolism. *Lancet*, 1990; 335:701-703.

17. Moinard C, et al. Involvement of glutamine, arginine, and polyamines in the action of ornithine alpha-ketoglutarate on macrophage functions in stressed rats. *J Leukoc Biol*, 2000; 67:834-840.

18. Kraemer TR, Burn BJ. Modulated mitogenic proliferation responsiveness of lymphocytes in whole blood cultures after a low-carotene diet and mixed carotenoid supplementation. *Am J Clin Nutr*. 1997; 65:871.

19. Serafini M. Dietary vitamin E and T cell-mediated function in the elderly: effectiveness and mechanism of action. *Int J Dev Neurosci*, 2000; 18:401j-410.

20. Lee CY, Man-Fan Wan J. Vitamin E supplementation improves cell-mediated immunity and oxidative stress of Asian men and women. *J Nutr*, 2000; 130:2932-2937.

Index

Medicine 99
Stomach cancer 18, 58, 88, 89, 132, 136, 141
  digestive tract tumors 132, 133
Stroke 44
Substantia nigra 21
Sugars 67, 110, 111
Sulfates 112
Sun. *See* Ultra-violet radiation and cancer; Skin cancer
Surgery 9, 131
Sweden 80
Syndrome X 29, 45
Syphilis 91

T

T-cell lymphocytes 159, 161
T-cell lymphotrophic virus 88, 92
Tamoxifen 134
Tannic acid 132
Tanning beds 80, 81
Tea 132, 133, 138
Testosterone 37, 38, 40, 41, 43
Teticular cancer 77
Thiamin 62
Thyroid cancer 59
Tobacco. *See* Smoking and cancer
Tobacco industry. *See* Smoking and cancer
Tocopherols 123, 140
Tocotrienols 123, 140
Trifluralin 57
Triglycerides 45
Trihalomethanes 71
Twinrix vaccine 89, 90
Twin studies 97

U

Ubiquinone. *See* Coenzyme Q10
Ultra-violet radiation and cancer 15, 16, 79–82, 123, 140, 166
Underwood, Eric 74
United States (US) 1, 3, 4, 5, 11, 14, 15, 24, 48, 54, 55, 58, 59, 64, 68, 71, 76, 81, 83, 88, 89, 92, 95, 97, 99, 108, 109, 110, 124, 125, 140, 141, 142, 161, 163, 165. *See also* America(n)
University of Southern California 30
University of Texas 29, 63
Urethral cancer 58
Urinary tract cancer 71
US Centers for Disease Control 56, 91
US Department of Agriculture 163
US Environmental Protection Agency 57, 76
US Food and Drug Administration 113
US National Academy of Sciences 54, 55, 97, 108
US National Cancer Institute 1, 4, 5, 11, 14, 29, 30, 68, 80, 105, 107, 108
US National Health and Nutrition Examination Survey 108, 109
US National Institutes of Health 80
US National Research Council 83, 97
US Recommended Dietary Allowances 109, 110, 148
US Recommended Dietary Allowances (RDA) 54, 55
Uterine cancer 10, 28, 29

V

Vanadium 54, 111
Vegetables 13, 14, 32, 64, 66, 74, 103, 105, 106, 107, 108, 109, 111, 115, 125, 131, 134, 137, 141, 142, 144

Dr. Michael Colgan

Michael Colgan, PhD, CCN, is an internationally renowned research scientist. He is acknowledged as one of the world's most popular scientific experts in nutrition, exercise and the inhibition of aging.

From 1971 to 1982, Dr. Colgan was a senior member of the Science Faculty of the University of Auckland, where he taught in Human Sciences and conducted research on aging and physical performance. Startling results of his early research convinced him to write his first book for the public, *Your Personal Vitamin Profile,* during his tenure as a visiting scholar at Rockefeller University in New York. This revolutionary book rapidly became a definitive guide for accurate, scientifically researched nutritional information.

From 1979 to 1998, Dr. Colgan was the Director and President of the Colgan Institute; now he serves as Chairman of the Board. The Colgan Institute has branches in the United States, Canada and Australasia. The Colgan Institute is a consulting, educational and research facility founded in 1979, primarily concerned with the effects of nutrition and exercise on athletic performance, aging and the prevention of degenerative disease. The Institute is also known for its revolutionary supplement programs, designed by Dr. Colgan, and only available directly through the Institute.

Dr. Colgan has served as a consultant to the US National Institute on Aging and to the New Zealand and Canadian Governments, as well as many corporations. His professional memberships include the American Academy of Anti-Aging Medicine, the American College of Sports Medicine, the New York Academy of Sciences, the British Society for Nutritional Medicine, and the International and American Associations of Clinical Nutritionists (IAACN). In 2002 Dr. Colgan was inducted into the Canadian Sports Nutrition Hall of Fame.

With a distinguished reputation for his expertise in sports nutrition, Dr. Colgan has advised hundreds of athletes of all abilities and ages throughout the world. These include track and field Olympians Donovan Bailey, Quincy Watts, Leroy Burrell, Steve Scott, Michelle Burrell, Meredith Rainey Valmon and Regina Jacobs; three-time world boxing champion Bobby Czyz; rowers Francis Reininger and Adrian Cassidy; powerlifter Rick Roberts; two-time world triathlon champion Julie Moss and world-class triathlete Brandyn Gray; shooting champion T'ai Erasmus; Australian heavyweight boxing champion Chris Sharpe; motorcross champion Danny Smith; and bodybuilding champions Lee Labrada, Lee Haney and Lenda Murray.

For more information on Dr. Colgan and the Colgan Institute, as well as information on Colgan Institute products, programs, and upcoming events, visit www.colganinstitute.com.